"Angelia Brigance weaves [...] aging mother with dementia. Along with a relatable story, she offers some practical tips to help families negotiate the emotional and sometimes overwhelming task of care-giving for their loved one experiencing a cognitive decline."

Naomi Bryant, ND
Chief Medical Officer
Naturo-Medica

"Angelia writes with simplicity and beauty. Her fictitious story is immediately relatable, especially for readers who have a loved one with dementia. Her practical, time-tested advice is woven into the story seamlessly, leaving the reader with love for the characters and tips for how to support someone suffering with dementia. A definite 'must-read.'"

Di Beals
Pastor
Canyon Creek Church

"As enjoyable as any novel, this book goes beyond and is a must-read for anyone with aging parents, relatives, or friends. In this compelling story, author Angelia Brigance has masterfully captured the subtle life-changes of the elderly, while gently, clearly, and compassionately educating her reader on how to lovingly go through this stage of life with them."

Dawn Jones
Best Selling Author
Top 7 Personality Challenges

FINDING
ROSE

A NOVEL

ANGELIA BRIGANCE

Made for Success
PUBLISHING

Made For Success Publishing
P.O. Box 1775 Issaquah, WA 98027
www.MadeForSuccessPublishing.com

Distributed by Made For Success Publishing
Editor: Katie Rios
Book Design: DeeDee Heathman
Executive Editor: Valerie Heathman

Library of Congress Cataloging-in-Publication data

Brigance, Angelia
Finding Rose: A Novel
p. cm.

ISBN: 978-1-64146-369-0 (PBK)
ISBN: 978-1-64146-370-6 (eBOOK)
LCCN: 2018961946

Dedicated to my husband who loves me and believes in me. Who encourages me to share my passion, stands by my side, and holds my hand throughout life. I am blessed and still, "can't live without you."

To my children, Gabrielle and Joshua, dreams do come true. My first dream was you. Your excitement and love through this book made my next dream a joy.

To my mom, the original Rose. Your impact on my life, your strength and love through life's challenges, gave me the vision to face whatever life brings.

Lastly, to the bouquet of Roses who have come and gone from my life, leaving a passion to walk through your memories and embrace them with you.

Chapter One

aureen found herself alone in a room that had oversized mahogany doors polished to a high sheen. She imagined that this room was where the elite came to have cocktail parties in the evening light, complete with big band music and dancing. She closed her eyes for a moment and took a deep breath. She felt the sun on her face and slowly opened her eyes.

The sun was shining brightly through a majestic window that filled one side of the room. The walls seemed to glimmer like gold as the afternoon sun bounced off them, filling the room with warmth. Down the halls, ornate furniture with lush gold fabric lined the walls with deep red drapes and pillows. Large vases bursting with fresh flowers filled the rooms with the smell of spring.

The room had held many parties and joyous celebrations, but not today. No, today the room had a somber effect with chairs lined up in rows to hold the many guests coming to pay their respects.

Dad had died suddenly just over two weeks ago. Maureen stood in the room alone to catch her breath, attempting to pull herself together before the guests arrived. At 5'5", Maureen was neither short nor tall. She was slender yet curvaceous, which she wasn't comfortable with. Maureen loved to hike in the mountains, and as a nurse, she got her steps in around the hospital, making it easy to keep her weight down. She wore her straight brown hair at shoulder length, and the cut followed the line of her jaw. Her deep-set eyes were brown with flecks of gold in them. Today she wore only light makeup, knowing it would probably be gone before the day was over. Mom had insisted. She looked out the window at the rolling green hills, taking advantage of fleeting moments of calm.

Maureen knew her dad would have loved knowing his memorial would be held here at the exclusive Los Angeles Country Club. Her brother Grant was a member. He and Dad were a lot alike. Grant Sr. was a doctor in private practice. He was only 5' 10", but he stood as if he were at least 6 feet tall. He always held himself with pride, and he had a laugh that could light up an entire room. Mom often said it was Dad's laughter she fell in love with. He did well enough for himself and his family. Mom never had to work, which allowed her to be the social butterfly. Where Dad had a warm intellect, Mom had a gregarious flare. They were the perfect balance.

At 6'1', Grant *did* stand tall. He looked up to Dad and inherited his drive for success, except his ambition was on steroids. He excelled in everything he did—from sports to academics, there seemed to be nothing he couldn't do. Dad would beam every time a new accolade was bestowed on him. He, of course, married the perfect model, Tiffany, and had a fairytale wedding.

Though Grant had a surfer look with sun-bleached hair and brown eyes, he had an impeccably shrewd mind. It made sense that he went into law; he could charm anyone. Dad was over the moon when Grant Jr. made partner in the firm. He was laser-focused, and he kept his sights on success.

Maureen sighed heavily thinking of her dad. Dad had played golf with Grant here just last month on his 80th birthday. She missed him and wondered if he had been as proud of her as he was of Grant.

As a child, Maureen loved to sit with her dad and read stories. They read adventures and mystery novels and went on walks hand in hand. Grant had come along when she was six years old (a surprise addition), and he changed everything. Dad was so excited to have a son. Maureen knew her dad loved her, but his face never shone as bright as when he looked at Grant. Maureen and her dad still shared secret looks and stories that Grant wasn't part of, but, over time, they had drifted apart.

When Maureen announced she was going to be a nurse, Dad was over the moon to have someone in the family following his footsteps in the medical field. The day she graduated, he brought her a bouquet of wildflowers and a stethoscope. Maureen reached up as if to touch the piece around her neck, remembering the joy she felt as if it was just yesterday. She wore it every day at work with pride. Graduation was *their* moment. Grant didn't like "medical talk"—blood and surgery details would send him flying out the door. Maureen had used this on more than one occasion to have time alone with her dad. She smiled remembering the time she and her dad were enthralled in a controversy about a new surgery technique at dinner and Grant ran out of the room just in time to throw up in the guest bathroom. After that, Mom declared no more shop talk at the table.

A year later, Maureen was gone. She had met and married her now husband of over 30 years, Steve, who had an opportunity to start a small construction company in the foothills outside of Seattle, Washington with a friend.

꧁

After what only felt like a few minutes, Maureen's quiet time was interrupted as family and friends began to fill the room. Her husband, Steve, walked in with their children and families following closely behind. Steve stood 5'10" with a strong build and gray-hazel eyes. He looked handsome with his salt and pepper hair cut short and neat. He was noticeably uncomfortable in the black suit and tie they had bought for the service, but he pulled it off nicely. Seattle was a more casual atmosphere than here in Beverly Hills, and they both preferred it.

Maureen's grandson, Nash, who had just turned one, ran down the aisle. To him, this was simply a new playground with lots of places to climb. His exuberance was a blessing. He had bright blue eyes that looked just like his great grandfather's. *Dad will live on through those eyes,* Maureen thought. Gabby, the eldest, ran after him. She had flown in for the service from Alaska, where her husband, Matt, was stationed in the Army. While Nash brought excitement, her arrival was always calming for Maureen. Motherhood agreed with her. She looked slim in her fitted black dress and heels. Her long brown hair was curled around her face, and she wore the diamond necklace her father had given her on her wedding day. Matt was helping her corral Nash. He threw Nash into the air and caught him, triggering a boisterous laugh.

Josh, the middle and only boy, was walking in with his younger sister, Grace. Josh was in college. Where Steve was uncomfortable in his suit, Josh filled it out and looked natural. He definitely knew clothes, having worked at Nordstrom for years to pay for school. He was studying personal training and nutrition and was an excellent ad for his future. Grace was a senior in high school. She was 5' 4", slim like her sister, with brown hair and green eyes the color of olives. Grace was a natural beauty. She was a social butterfly like her grandmother, Rose.

The whole clan sat down with Maureen, with Steve at her side and the children in the row behind them. Steve took her hand and gave it a squeeze. He was her strength.

Rose entered the room with the style and elegance of a classic movie star. She wore a black knee length dress with a single strand of pearls. Her short, light brown hair had a curl that framed her face under her hat—Mom's signature accessory. The hat she chose today was black linen with a wide brim, worn low on one side. Black netting with small pearls accented the low slope of the hat. She stood at the door with her head down, slowly raising it until you could see her light green eyes. A small drop of the black netting from the hat almost met her eyes. She looked beautiful. She was quiet and reserved—at least for the moment—willing herself to be strong.

Grant walked up next to Mom in his custom back suit and took her arm to sit her down so the memorial could begin. Tiffany followed, looking as if she had walked straight out of a fashion show, strutting down the runway. Maureen silently groaned watching her. The rest of the guests were filtering in and taking seats. Maureen saw family, friends, patients, and colleagues from Dad's former practice entering to honor him. She nodded to a few as they sat down around her. The burial had already taken place earlier that day with only family and close friends.

Grant had center stage for the service. He spoke eloquently about Dad, his practice, and his love of golf. The room was filled to the brim, and Grant was captivating. He even managed to weave in a few stories about Maureen and Mom into the mix. The mood was light with just enough somber undertones to be respectful. Maureen could picture Grant talking in front of a jury, taking them on a journey. He and Dad had that in common. Dad was a storyteller. He was always running behind at the office because he was busy sharing life with his patients. It was precisely why people were willing to wait to see him.

Grant finished, and their parents' long-time pastor came up to the front to speak and share a bit more before it was over. Maureen loved hearing these stories about her dad. They involved the whole family and brought back great memories. The memorial concluded with both laughter and tears; a beautiful celebration of an amazing life.

Guests stopped by Rose, Maureen, and Grant to share their sympathy and quick memories before going out onto the patio for refreshments. Rose held Maureen's hand and carried on a light conversation. Occasionally, Rose seemed overwhelmed and forgot the name of a longtime friend or got mixed up by the story they were telling. "She's exhausted," Maureen would explain. Maureen would often find Rose looking past the crowd at Dad's portrait—which was on a gilded stand at the front of the room—as if to say, "Where are you? I need you." Maureen's heart broke a bit more. Soon, they were finally able to go outside and enjoy some of the warm afternoon air.

Nash was running through the crowd laughing, and Gabby was trying to keep him "proper" and safe in an outdoor patio where the golf course was a temptation. Matt, Josh, and Grace were teaming up to help, but Nash looked like he was winning. He ran up to Maureen and gave her his signal for "up." Maureen picked him up and cuddled with him. It was a play to get to the grass, but she didn't care. She couldn't wait to hear him call her "GiGi"—the grandma name she had chosen when Gabby first announced she was expecting. Steve walked up, and Nash said "Papa," leaving Maureen to try "up" with another. Maureen stood for a moment watching them, grateful to have them nearby. Gabby met her eyes, checking in. She knew how hard the day had been already. Maureen smiled at Gabby, letting her know she was fine.

The morning had been tough. Mom had been scattered, and they were all rushed. Rose couldn't find her pearls, and she just *had* to have them. They were a gift from Dad for their 50th wedding anniversary. They had looked everywhere. Finally, Maureen found them in the *silverware drawer*. It was certainly odd, but Mom blamed it on the housekeeper, and there was no time to ponder. Mom had notes up all throughout the house so she wouldn't forget anything. The stress from dad being gone left her feeling disorganized, to say the least. She seemed a little off to Maureen, but in the end, it made sense. She and Dad had been together for so long that standing on her own again would take some time. They were finally ready just as the limousine Grant had ordered showed up to take them to the cemetery.

Now, hours later, in the midst of the crowd, Rose seemed more at home. She loved to entertain guests, and this reception was her stage. She chatted and moved through the crowd. As the crowd thinned, Maureen saw her standing in front of the portrait of Grant, looking at it as if he were really there. A small group was nearby talking with Grant Jr. and Tiffany. Maureen's family was seated at a nearby table, Nash having finally given up and fallen asleep in Matt's arms.

Rose began to walk away from the portrait, then suddenly turned around. She looked over her shoulder, and in her best Ingrid Bergman voice, said, "Kiss me, kiss me as if it were the last time." The guests around Grant let out a small gasp, while the family just rolled their eyes. It was from *Casablanca*, Mom and Dad's favorite movie. They shared lines from that movie all through their marriage as if it were their own life. Grant explained his mom's dramatic flair and the rest of the group chuckled. She could make a grand entrance—or exit—anywhere.

Chapter Two

The days Maureen had spent at Mom's had been bittersweet. Old memories, old friends, and family had filled the few days they had spent together. They laughed and cried; sometimes at the same things. Memories had a funny way of doing that. Maureen felt melancholy as she packed her bag knowing Mom would be alone in a house full of memories. Saying goodbye to Mom gave Maureen a twinge of sadness and guilt.

The morning they left, Mom insisted on making breakfast for everyone. On the menu were pancakes, eggs, and crispy bacon. Everything was going smoothly until smoke began pouring out of the oven. In the excitement and hustle of the morning, Mom forgot that the bacon was in the oven and it was burning. It looked more like ashes when Maureen opened the oven.

Maureen took care of the mess, then spent time calming Mom down—who was deeply upset that she had ruined breakfast. Gabby and Josh fanned the smoke detectors to get them to stop whaling, while Steve and Matt opened the doors and windows. Nash sat in his high chair eating pancakes and syrup, watching the excitement with wide eyes. He waved his arms at everyone, but they weren't quite sure if he was just enjoying himself or signaling for help. Grace was still getting ready upstairs and hadn't even heard the alarm. The incident took the edge off of everyone. Later, as they ate their pancakes and eggs around the kitchen table, laughter and stories of past cooking disasters filled the air.

Grant stopped by before they left for the airport to go over the details of the plan. The "plan" was to move Mom up to Washington into her own place in several months, giving her time to sort through her things. Grant was busy putting the estate in order so he could sell the house, and after it sold, Mom would fly to Seattle to start her new adventure.

Change, even good change, is hard. However, Maureen knew that having her mom close to her was important. Grant and Tiffany were too busy with their own lives.

◆

Maureen and Steve said goodbye to Gabby, Matt, and Nash after going through security to fly home. Their flight was on the other side of the airport, and they were running late. The rest of the family headed toward their gate. They stopped at Starbucks for drinks and snacks—a travel ritual. A skinny vanilla latte, Americano, and two Frappuccinos. It was easy to guess who drank what. Maureen was starting to relax, and Steve took her hand as they strolled along.

After settling in at the gate, Maureen heard her and Steve's name called at the customer service desk. Steve got up to check on it, and Maureen took a moment to watch Grace and Josh. They were both on their phones, talking about something posted on Instagram. She smiled watching them. Steve returned and said they had changed their seats. "No big deal. The kids are still next to each other."

A few minutes later, the loudspeaker announced boarding. "Boarding for flight 4426 to Seattle is now beginning. Those with special priority boarding and first-class seats are welcome to begin." Maureen was confused when Steve stood up.

"Honey, it will be a bit. Sit down and relax."

"Nope, *we* are boarding *now*," Steve smiled and gave her the new boarding pass. He had changed their tickets to first class! Maureen couldn't believe her eyes. She had never ridden in first class, and couldn't imagine what had made Steve do it. "I thought you needed this," he said matter-of-factly and took her hand. Josh and Grace complained that they didn't get to sit in first class, but smiled at them as they disappeared down the walkway. Several minutes later, Josh and Grace passed them on their way to their seats. Glasses of wine and a plate of cheese and fruit were already on their table. They looked happy and relaxed.

That would be the last time Maureen would relax for quite some time.

It started a few days after returning home. At first, Rose called each evening. She didn't really have anything to talk about; she just wanted to hear Maureen's voice. "She's lonely," Maureen told Steve one evening in bed after the latest call.

Then the calls became more frequent. Maureen's phone would go off several times a day. It interrupted work, church, and sleep.

"The house is overwhelming her. She needs help sorting through everything. I thought you were going to help her with this? You are there Grant, please. I need you to help her," Maureen begged and scolded Grant at the same time.

"She just wants attention. She's fine," Grant responded.

"Grant, please! Dad was at her side all the time, and she is alone now. Please get her some help. If you can't do it yourself, you need to find someone who can." Maureen's voice raised more than she had expected, and Grant decided it would be better to concede.

"Fine, OK. First thing in the morning I will call and have my secretary hire a company to help her."

"Thank you, Grant," Maureen hung up the phone and sighed. She hoped it would be enough.

Grant did as he promised, and an agency came to help Rose the next afternoon. The calls lessened during the day, giving Maureen a break and allowing her to concentrate at work. Night, however, was a different story.

Rose kept calling, worried that "the staff Grant had sent were stealing from her." They were nice, but she was concerned about the family heirlooms and told Maureen she was hiding some things to keep them safe. Maureen would spend time calming Mom down and reassuring her. She encouraged her to give things to Grant to ship if she was worried or pack them at night. None of it seemed to be a real threat, and Maureen wondered if Grant were right and she just wanted attention. To be safe, she called Grant and asked him to go over to check on Mom and see how the house was going. He was busy with an upcoming trial, so he begrudgingly agreed to send Tiffany. *A lot of help she'll be,* Maureen thought, but it was the best she was going to get right now.

Maureen wasn't ready for what came next. Mom had called and casually mentioned the nice policemen that had been over earlier in the day. Alarmed, Maureen asked, "Why? What happened Mom? Are you OK?"

"Yes honey, everything is fine. I thought I heard something in the garage, so they came over to check it out. It turned out it was nothing. They were so kind and handsome."

A few days later, it was the fire department. It seemed that the smoke detector batteries were low, and she thought an alarm was going off—although she couldn't figure out why. "They changed the battery, and all was well."

"Mom," Maureen explained, "you can't call the police or fire department unless it's an emergency."

"Oh, it was. Honey, the sound was awful!"

Maureen groaned. Mom was high maintenance. How did Dad do it?

Even so, Maureen got into a routine. Days were quiet, for the most part, and then the night would come with some sort of extravagant story. Mom wasn't calling 911 anymore, but the washer and dryer broke, and it seemed things were always missing. Each night when the phone rang, Maureen poured herself a glass of wine and listened. It was all she could do. Tonight, the call was about her hats.

"How will I get them to Washington safely? I need hat boxes. They will have to be packed special. One might be missing…"

Once Maureen hung up after an hour or more of conversation, she would recant the stories to Steve and Grace. It had become their nighttime entertainment.

Maureen checked her phone when she went on her lunch break at work. It had been a long day on the surgical ward. She needed a break. She always cringed a bit as she turned on her phone, worried that Mom might have had another emergency. She had been better during the day, but she was known for surprises. Maureen's heart raced when she saw she had a message from Grant. He usually didn't initiate calls, especially since Dad had passed.

"Call me when you get this. Thanks." That was the whole message. *Well, that doesn't help,* she thought as she called him back. His secretary answered the call and asked her to wait. Time seemed to stop as she waited for Grant to get to the phone. "We have to do something about Mom," were his first words. No "Hello," or "Sorry to worry you," just, "We have to do something about Mom."

It seemed that Mom had been causing a ruckus. Grant went on to describe her calls to Tiffany and him for "ridiculous" things at all hours. Maureen laughed at that statement, thinking of her nightly calls with Mom. "I don't have time for this," Grant went on. "Do you know she has called 911 six times in the last three weeks? Now they call me!" This surprised Maureen as Mom hadn't mentioned it in her calls. She had mentioned the nice people that had been helping her lately. Had these "people" been the police?

"She has to stop. I know the police chief in town, and he called me himself. She could get in trouble Maureen. What are we going to do?" Grant sounded angry.

"Grant, I am thousands of miles away. I understand that there is a lot left to do in the house, the estate isn't closed, and the house isn't ready to even be put on the market yet. But what do you want *me* to do?" *He needs to step up,* Maureen thought. *Deal with it.*

What she wasn't prepared for was his solution.

"Mom wants more attention than Tiffany and I can give her," He started. Maureen could hear the closing argument in his voice, so she sat up to pay close attention. He had obviously come up with a new "plan" and was going to lay it out for her. She held her breath.

"The estate will be closed in a few months. Mom is not cooperating with the organizers to get the house packed. I need to have professionals come in to do repairs before the sale. She needs to be out of the house *now*," pausing as he took a quick breath. "The plan was always for Mom to move to Washington. The only difference is she needs to move now." The closing argument hit home, and Grant was silent. So was Maureen.

Grant waited for the response. He had answers to all expected questions.

"When?"

"Within a week. I can get her packed and ready with her essentials."

"How?"

"You can fly here and then fly back together. She can take more on the plane that way and would be less likely to argue about it."

"Where?"

"We can't purchase a new home for her until the estate closes and we can sell the house. She can stay with you."

"Excuse me?!" Maureen exclaimed. Mom's nightly calls were one thing, but having her at the house 24/7 for what could be months was going to be a tall order. It made her weary just thinking about it. "It makes sense Maureen. She can get the attention she wants and will calm down. Maureen, Mom wants to be near you." He pulled a heartstring, and she knew he knew it.

"Grant, I am going to have to talk to Steve about it tonight. We don't even have a bedroom for her. Where would she sleep? All we have is the basement, and it is *not* finished… I have to go."

Maureen hung up without saying goodbye. Her mind was racing with what to do and how she would approach Steve that night. Her lunch was in front of her, but she couldn't eat. She sat quietly for a few minutes before going back to finish her shift.

⌇

Steve sensed Maureen's mood as soon as he came into the house. *Hmmm,* he thought, *who has done what?* He greeted her with a quick kiss and went into their room to get cleaned up for dinner. She had looked at him and smiled, but her eyes spoke what she didn't have to: she was worried. He could tell she was trying to sort something out in her mind, and Steve knew that she would talk when she was ready.

Dinner was pleasant and simple. Pasta and salad—Grace's favorite. Prom was coming up soon, and Grace happily rambled on about her plans with her date, Brandon. Maureen chimed in, but Steve could see she wasn't really listening. Grace cleaned up after dinner, still talking about dresses and shoes. She bounced up to her room to call friends, and hopefully, do homework.

"Are you ready to talk?" Steve asked cautiously. Maureen looked up from her chair at Steve. "I think we may need a drink for this one," she said quietly as she moved into her favorite chair in the front room. Steve poured them each a whiskey and ginger ale. He handed one to her and sat in his chair next to her.

"OK, here it goes," Maureen said, taking a sip of her drink. She told Steve everything that Grant had said that day. All the things Mom was doing and the calls to the police. "I have been racking my brain all day, and I just don't see any options. If she stays there, who knows what she will do next. If she comes here... How?"

Steve listened and nodded as Maureen let it all out. He needed that drink indeed. Watching her as she spoke, he could see the pain she was in. He knew the only way they could make it work. It would cost them, but he couldn't stand to see Maureen hurting. Steve took the last sip of his drink and offered up the basement. It would need a lot of work in a short amount of time, but he would get it done. It would also deplete most of their Italian vacation fund. They had been saving for this trip for nearly two years and planned to take it the year after Grace graduated.

"Are you sure?" Maureen had tears in her eyes. She knew what the trip meant and the sacrifice he was making.

"Happy wife, happy life," he said and smiled.

Maureen came over and sat on Steve's lap. He held her in his strong arms, and she felt herself melt into this man who loved her well. Life was about to get interesting.

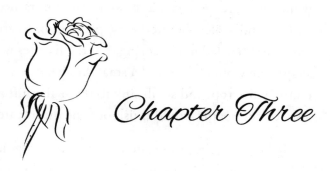

Chapter Three

Maureen would be going down to pick up Rose in about a week, and Steve still had a lot to do. In its current state, the basement was just that: an unfinished room with exposed walls, concrete floors and a door to the side of the house. Thankfully, a single ceiling light and a set of small windows brightened up the otherwise dark space.

As he neared the bottom of the steps, Steve remembered that the basement already had a small full bathroom with a shower. *Thank God for small favors*, he thought, taking it all in and getting a feel for the work he would have to do.

Steve spent the next couple of hours sketching out the plans for the room, taking inventory of all that needed to be done. The walls would have to be insulated and sealed with drywall, then textured and painted—ceiling included. The ceiling fixture would need to be replaced to bring in more light. He would have to check all the electrical outlets, and potentially add a couple more. The windows needed to be reframed, and window sills would need to be added. A closet would have to be created as well. The floors needed to be treated and sealed before being padded and carpeted. The bathroom needed new flooring, but the fixtures were in good shape. He would also build a small kitchenette with a refrigerator, stove top, and small sink to the makeshift studio, and a set of cupboards would finish out the dining area.

If he was going to create a room, he was going to do it right. He made his list of what he was going to need and headed down to Home Depot to get supplies.

It took Steve the better part of two hours to get everything together at the store. Three utility carts precariously balanced the variety of materials he was going to need as he quietly checked over his lists and moved about the store. He was a regular there, so the pro desk was being helpful by taking away carts as he filled them and held them in the front.

As he was filling the third cart with some last-minute add-ons, Steve saw another contractor he occasionally worked with, Arash. Steve liked working with Arash. He was smart, had a strong work ethic, and was wildly creative.

Arash was watching Steve with amusement. "Are you playing a game of Tetris? That stack looks like it could topple over at any minute."

Steve looked up and laughed. "Yeah, I guess so. I didn't want to have to get another cart. This is my third one."

"What's the job?" Arash inquired.

"Turning my unfinished basement into a place where my mother-in-law can stay for a few months; she'll be there until her house sells in LA. I have about a week to get it all done," Steve said as he ran his hand through his hair and shook his head. "I have no idea how I am going to get it done."

"Been there, done that. We did the same thing for my mother-in-law."

"You did? How long did she stay?" Steve looked hopeful.

"Well, at the last count it has been 22 years. Sorry man, wish I had better news for you. Hey, I have a couple of days open right now. Why don't I come over and help you out? We need to stick together in these situations." Arash started to push the cart to the desk. He looked back at Steve, who hadn't blinked or moved a muscle. "It'll be OK man. Now come on and tell me what you have planned."

Steve shook the worry from his mind and caught up with Arash, sharing his ideas for the room. Arash added a few ideas of his own, and they made plans to start the next morning, giving Steve a bit of time to prep. Once the truck was loaded and he was driving home, Steve contemplated what it would be like having Rose at the house and how long she might actually stay.

The next morning, the two men got started in the basement. Steve had spent the previous day prepping walls and floors, putting in three additional electrical outlets and laying down the rudiments for the kitchen. He was already sore, and the hard work had yet to begin. Josh came down to help the "old men" with the heavy lifting and quickly decided that construction work was harder than the gym. Grace popped in with drinks, lunch, and snacks since Maureen was at work.

At the end of day one, they amazed themselves with all they had accomplished. The shell of the room was complete, except for paint. The bathroom floor had been replaced, and the kitchenette had a countertop and cabinets. All three men were covered in sweat and dust, smiles of satisfaction spreading across their worn-out faces.

Arash left to head home, and Josh and Steve each took long, hot showers. Clean, yet exhausted, they ate the dinner Grace had left for them before getting comfortable and passing out in the front room watching TV. When Maureen got home from work, she nudged them to go to their rooms. It didn't take a whole lot of convincing to get them off the couch and into their own beds. It wasn't late, but they had put in a full days' work and needed some rest before another big day.

Steve buried himself in the basement for the next several days. Josh helped when he could, and a few of Steve's friends stopped by and lent a hand after Arash went on to his own projects. Maureen went out with Grace and bought furniture and décor to make the room feel comfortable and cozy. Grace was going to decorate the room while Maureen was picking up Rose—time was running out.

Steve put the finishing touches on the room the night before Maureen left for California. The furniture had arrived—some in boxes—and Josh would help get it together while Grace decorated. Gabby had ordered some special pieces for the room as well. The basement conversion had become a family project for Rose. Although Grace and Josh had expressed their willingness to move to the basement several times that week as they saw it take shape, Maureen and Steve thanked them for their sacrifice and said "no."

⤺

The morning flight to LAX was uneventful, and Maureen took a shuttle to the house. They were flying back together the next afternoon, and she had no idea what she was walking into.

Rose was excited to see her arrive, and Maureen was pleasantly surprised by the condition of the house. The company Grant had hired was doing a great job. The knick-knacks and personal items that seemed to be tucked away in every corner of the house had been packed, and the house looked simple with clean lines. After being pared down, the furniture had been moved to show off the best features of the house and created an inviting cohesiveness from room to room. Vases were out in each room, ready to be filled with fresh flowers before the house started to show. The garage was the staging area for the move, and boxes were stacked against the walls.

Rose had prepared a small meal for them to share when Maureen arrived. They sat at the table, enjoying a cup of tea and slices of warm banana bread with cream cheese. "No fire alarms?" Maureen teased her mom as they ate.

"Heavens no. I stayed right here and watched it. Melts in your mouth, doesn't it?"

"It sure does Mom."

Rose grinned, happy to see her eldest enjoying the bread. The day passed quickly. There were suitcases that needed to be packed and last-minute questions from the staff working in the house. Some were there fixing appliances and electrical, while others were painting rooms with fresh white paint.

Mom had always been into color. Each room had its own color scheme, and she changed it on a whim several times over the years. Maureen liked color as well and was a little sad to see all of it go. She would have liked more time to wander through the house and reminisce, but there were too many things to do before their morning flight back home. Mom had to consolidate down to four bags for the flight, not including the carry on. That may have seemed like a lot, but Mom was a clothes hound. On top of that, she loved hats and jewelry. She wasn't about to leave them behind.

Grant and Tiffany brought over Chinese take-out for dinner from Mom's favorite restaurant. Maureen, Grant, and Rose ate with chopsticks, as they always had. They tried to convince Tiffany to give it a try, but she refused. She didn't like anything that could be messy. Grant was relaxed, cracking jokes and playing around. Maureen loved when her brother was in this mood. Sometimes she thought he lost it, but on occasion, he let it slip out and let his guard down. It definitely made the evening easier.

In the morning, Maureen and Rose enjoyed a coffee and the last of the banana bread. They took a walk through the neighborhood and said goodbye to some of Mom's closest friends. Grant came back to the house to load up the van he had rented. The driver would help get the luggage all the way to check in. That was a true blessing. Maureen was sure his secretary had thought of the gesture, and she was happy for it. They had four extra-large violet suitcases—two filled with hats, jewelry and make-up and two filed with clothes—ready to go. Maureen was certain they were over the 50-pound limit, but she couldn't get Rose to leave anything else behind. In the end, she let her fill them up as much as she could.

The ride to the airport was slow in the mid-morning traffic, but they still moved along nicely and arrived fairly quickly. The driver took care of the luggage and walked with them to the ticket counter to check in the bags. As she thought, all were well over 50 pounds. They paid the fees and went off to head through security.

Maureen was relieved that the last few days had gone relatively painlessly. One chapter was closed, more or less, and another about to open. Maureen was a little nervous to head home and see what life would be like for each of them.

⚘

As soon as she walked in the house, Maureen was greeted by the smell of fresh paint and flowers. Grace had a huge bouquet on the counter filled with breathtaking spring flowers from Pike's Market. It was a lovely surprise.

"Mom, do you want to see your room?" Maureen hadn't seen it since it had been finished, so she was as excited as she hoped Mom would be to see it.

"Yes of course!" Rose seemed happy, and Maureen felt like maybe she really did just need some TLC. They walked down the few stairs to the basement and opened the door.

The room was so much more than Maureen could have hoped or dreamed. Steve had painted the main walls a soft grey with white trim, and the bedroom area had a muted violet hue to bring in some color for Mom. Grace had the bed made with a floral print bedspread with violet and pink roses, throw pillows of varied shades of pink and violet and a cream-colored bed skirt. On one side of the bed stood a white-washed night stand with a small vase of silk roses, and on the other, a soft violet chair and ottoman. A silver standing lamp with crystals was tucked in behind the chair, and a lace divider gave the area some privacy.

A dark grey loveseat, a matching violet chair and ottoman, and white end tables finished off the small living space. There was a television on the wall across from the loveseat so Rose could watch some of her favorite shows. The kitchenette had a small white table with two chairs, already set with a variety of plates, glasses, and stemware they had found at Home Goods. Floral dish towels lay on the counter below a set of rose-colored mugs hung from under the cupboards. On the walls, intermixed with floral prints, were pictures of the family that Gabby had ordered and Grace framed in white wood frames. The bath was filled with pastel towels, lavender soap, and a shower curtain that matched the bedspread.

All of it was lovely. The part of the room that Steve was most proud of was the closet. It looked like a professional company like California Closets had come in and built it out with varied levels for long and short clothes. Drawers were built in, so a dresser wouldn't be needed. In an effort to make Mom feel seen and known, Steve built an area of the closet just for her hats. There were several slots to neatly tuck some of them away and another area for hat boxes. Steve had genuinely thought of everything.

Maureen gave Steve a hug and a kiss and watched as Rose looked around the room. He put his arm around Maureen as she rested her head on his shoulder. They went back upstairs and left Rose and Grace sitting on the couch talking.

Later, Steve hauled the suitcases downstairs. Rose gave him a kiss on the cheek and thanked him for all he had done, and Grace spent the evening helping Rose start to settle in.

Maureen had an early shift the next morning. She left with the house still dark and quiet.

⤐

Rose woke up and looked around the room, a little confused as to where she had just slept. She lay there for a moment until she remembered the move. She rolled over to look at her nightstand and her picture of Grant. It had always been on her nightstand, and it was the first thing she had put out when they unpacked the night before. "Here's looking at you kid," she whispered to him.

Rose spent the morning in her room. She put away more clothes and arranged her jewelry and hats. She made a cup of tea and toast and sat down at the small white table. The TV remote was sitting on the table, so she picked it up and started pushing buttons. The television wouldn't turn on, so she decided to go for a walk instead.

She picked up her phone and purse and went upstairs. The house was quiet. Everyone was gone for the day at work or school. Rose opened the front door and turned right at the sidewalk, just like she did at home. She talked with a few folks who were outside as she went along, enjoying herself along the winding road. She loved fresh air.

After walking for quite some time, Rose thought she would head home for some lunch. However, when she turned around and started walking back, she was uneasy. She wasn't exactly sure where she was and if she knew how to get back home. Everything looked different. She walked for a long while, looking for something or someone familiar.

Josh happened to be driving home from his classes and saw Rose walking slowly a mile or more from home. He pulled over on the street in front of her and got out.

"Grandma Rose, let me give you a ride home. You walked a long way. You must be tired!"

Relieved, Rose answered, "Oh Josh, yes, I would love a ride back. Guess I went farther than I planned. It is such a nice day outside." She hopped in Josh's car, and they were home in just a few minutes. Rose realized that even in the short distance, she hadn't known how to get back—but she was keeping that to herself.

Once home, Rose prepared lunch for the both of them while he fixed the television in her room. It took a few minutes for him to figure out which buttons she had pressed; he had never seen the screen it was on before. He then showed her how to use the remote, telling her which buttons were to turn on the system and which were for changing the channels and sound.

They ate lunch together, and she asked about his classes. She told him stories of when he was a young boy that he hadn't heard before. He had to leave to head off to work, so Rose sat on the loveseat to watch TV. She was tired after her morning adventure. She found an old movie on AMC, and it brought back memories of her and Grant dating. She fell asleep peacefully with him on her mind.

The afternoon was busy as Grace and her friends were planning for prom and graduation. Rose sat at the kitchen table upstairs, listening to the girls and looking at dresses on their computers. Fashion was one of Rose's favorite things. They talked about hair, makeup, jewelry and all the things Rose loved. They listened to her tell stories of her own prom and the many galas she had attended. Maureen arrived home from work and joined in as well.

The girls went upstairs when Maureen and Rose started dinner. They still had finals to study for, although both women knew that wasn't going to happen. The day had gone well, as far as Maureen knew. She had enjoyed sharing the kitchen with her mom cooking dinner. It was a peaceful way to spend time together.

Rose went to her room soon after dinner to watch TV. She called Steve down to fix the television as she had "hit some button" and it wouldn't go on. He had it on again quickly and showed her how to use the remote again. "Thank you, Steve. This darn thing has too many buttons on it, and

I can never get the right one," Rose explained. She didn't mention that Josh had fixed it earlier in the day.

Rose had gotten into a routine at her old home, and she was building the same here in Washington. Each morning she had toast and tea in her room, followed by a walk. She stayed on the same route each day, much shorter than her first adventure, and made it back home on her own. She kept an old envelope in her purse from a past Mother's Day card that had Maureen's address on it, just in case she got lost. She used it on occasion, showing the address to a neighbor who then pointed her in the right direction.

Once she was back at the house, she called Maureen, who would be taking a break at work at that time and would have a brief conversation. Lunch usually followed, some-times with Josh or Grace, who loved having a meal made for them. They had started to leave her reminder notes for when they would be home, as she had previously made them lunch—forgetting they wouldn't be home—and been upset by their absence. This seemed to work well for them. Rose had her "shows" in the afternoon and would watch television in her room, take a short nap, then come upstairs as the family began to gather in the early evening.

Occasionally, Rose had started dinner or tried to help with tidying up in the house. It was not always a success. On more than one occasion Rose had overflowed a sink, ruined a dish in the dishwasher by putting items on the bottom shelf that were *top shelf safe only* (causing them to melt), and forgot something cooking on the stove. Most of the time, Rose would clean up the water and throw away the dish or food before anyone saw her mistake. She was deeply embarrassed by the situations, and couldn't believe her bad luck. *Everything is different at this house,* Rose thought. *Why were things so complicated?* There were times when someone would walk in while Rose was in the middle of cleaning up the evidence, but they all figured it would take time for her to get used to things and no one really thought much more about it.

Rose loved to shop, and walked to a local store every Wednesday to pick up small things for the house and browse around at the gift shop. The store had local produce and a cheese counter that served fresh mozzarella, goat cheese, and feta. Local honey and chocolate were store specialties as well. In the gift shop, there were unique necklaces and earrings made by a local artist, which always caught her eye. The shop owner, Debbie, had gotten to know Rose over the past few weeks and made sure to have taste tests for her to enjoy when she arrived.

"Good morning Rose," Debbie said over the cheese counter where she had cut a few thin slices of a new cheddar they were featuring. "I have something new for you to taste today." She handed Rose the sample and came around the counter to see what Rose thought.

"It is lovely, Debbie. A little sharp to start with a creaminess at the end. We will have to have some of this for tonight's tacos." Debbie sliced about a pound and set it aside for her, knowing she would look around for a while before heading out. Rose picked up a few more items for dinner and went to check out, but she quickly realized she didn't have her purse. She was frantic and began looking all over the store. She never left the house without her purse.

"Rose, don't worry. I will keep an eye out for it, but I didn't remember seeing it when you came in. Why don't you look at home? You can owe me for the groceries. No problem. I will see you next week." Debbie's voice was kind and helpful. It wasn't the first time Rose had forgotten her purse. Maureen was also a regular, so she took care of it whenever she came in.

"Thank you, Debbie. I always have my purse with me. I just... I don't understand what happened." Rose left the store with the groceries and walked home, all the while trying to remember how she had gone out without her purse. Upon arriving home, Rose saw her purse waiting for her on the nightstand in her room. "That's what happened," she mumbled to herself. "I always have my purse next to the door. The cleaning lady was here this morning; I bet she moved it. She is always moving my stuff around, and I can't find anything."

Chapter Four

Grant had called Maureen occasionally over the months to ask questions and get information from Rose as he settled the estate and looked at offers from potential buyers. "I don't get it. Mom was good at home. She kept everything in order and was never late, but the mess I have on my hands right now is... is unimaginable," Grant started. "Bills are late—I mean really late. On top of the debt she racked up?! I bet Dad didn't even know."

"Now Grant, you know Dad would never deny her anything and there is nothing we can do now. Just pay what she owes, and let's be done with it." Maureen was always the practical big sister. "I am done, Maureen. The estate should have been closed already. The time it is taking is ridiculous.," Grant retorted.

He sighed. "It is just *way* more than I expected. She was giving money to at least a dozen charities and fundraisers every month. I hope the offer on the house coming in tomorrow is a good one. If it is, I can at least get these things paid off. That should leave Mom with a modest amount to live on."

Maureen could hear the concern in his voice—something she was not used to hearing. "At least we have a handle on it now, Grant. Let's hope tomorrow brings good news."

The offer on the house came in the next afternoon, and thankfully it was in the range—although it was on the lower end—of what Grant had hoped to get. He signed it off and called Maureen and Rose with the good news.

"Hello, Gr—"

"We are in escrow," he shared excitedly, cutting off Maureen before she could get any further.

"That's great news! Let me get Mom for you."

She brought the phone to Rose in her room. Rose was curled up on her couch watching an AMC movie with a glass of wine nibbling on cheese and crackers. She looked happy. "Mom, Mom... Grant has good news for you," Maureen smiled as she handed the phone to Rose. She watched her mother's face fall as Grant told her the news. Rose forced a smile as she looked at Maureen.

"Thank you, Grant. Your father would be proud. Yes, I understand. We will go down to sign final papers in a couple of weeks and make decisions on the rest of my things. Here, talk to your sister. You two make the arrangements." Rose handed back the phone to Maureen and focused on the movie. It was like losing her husband all over again. Maureen took the phone and headed back upstairs to work out details with Grant. She stopped at the door and looked back at her mother. She was in the same position on the couch, but her smile was replaced by slow falling tears. It broke Maureen's heart.

❧

In the two weeks that followed, there was a lot of discussion about furniture, art, and all the boxes that were now tucked away in a storage unit near the house. Rose put on a determined face and went along with the plans. The new owners liked some of the pieces of furniture left behind, so with Rose's permission, Grant added them to the sale of the house. He also arranged an estate sale for the other furniture and belongings that Rose would not be taking with her. After watching her mom when she heard about the sale of the house, Maureen was worried about the estate sale and the toll it would have on her. However, in typical Rose fashion, she would surprise them all.

They flew into town on a Thursday night and stayed at the Carlyle Inn. Rose loved the Carlyle. It reminded her of the old movies she loved to watch. The hotel theme was black and white with a definite Jazz flare. The music of Benny Good-man, Ella Fitzgerald, and Dean Martin could be heard softly overhead as you walked the halls. Rose and Grant Sr. had attended many events there over the years. It was also their local getaway when they wanted a romantic weekend. It had been a few years since she had last been there, but she felt right at home. Rose hummed to the music as they made their way to the room.

The next day, Rose and Maureen went through the storage unit, deciding what items *had* to stay in the family and what could go to the estate sale. Grant had hired help to move things back to the house for the sale. They packed things in a truck as soon as they heard a "yes, it can go," so Rose couldn't change her mind. In the end, Rose was letting go of more than either Grant or Maureen would have imagined. She kept a few pieces of art that she wanted to take with her or give away to someone special. A few mementos that Grant Sr. had given her over the years were to go home with her, as well as any jewelry or hats that she hadn't been able to take the first time. Maureen had a few items she wanted, and Grant kept some of his father's things as well. When the truck left, the storage unit was empty. The belongings they were keeping were packed into the back of Grant's Denali SUV.

They were exhausted by the time they got back to their room, but the sun was still shining and felt warm and invit-ing. Maureen and Rose sat in lounge chairs on their deck with a glass of iced tea, overlooking the pool and enjoying the sunshine. The sun relaxed them, and they both fell asleep for a while. Startled, they both jumped at the sound of the phone.

"Hello?" Maureen answered.

"Hello. We have reservations at Spago at 7. We'll pick you up at 6:45." It was Tiffany.

"Oh yeah, Grant told me that this morning. Glad you called." Maureen looked at her watch; it was nearly 5. "Guess we should start thinking about getting ready. We'll meet you downstairs at 6:45. Thank you again for the reminder."

"Great. We will be out front then. Bye." Maureen laughed to herself. Tiffany was a woman of few words. She was famished and was looking forward to dinner.

❧

Dinner was wonderful. Grant and Tiffany had a window table reserved, and the lights of the city twinkled at them. Grant engaged Rose in conversation about her experiences since moving in with Maureen, and she was happy to tell him. In between stories they discussed the estate sale the next morning.

"Mom, are you sure you want to be there?" Grant asked, worried that it might be too much for her.

"Oh yes, Grant. Who else can tell the stories behind all the items? They may want to know their history you know."

Rose was smiling and serious all at once. It was her way of saying goodbye.

◦◦

The estate sale started early. Grant had arranged for a company to manage the day, but Rose wanted to be there. Maureen wasn't sure how she would handle her possessions being sold to strangers, but it was her mother's things after all, and she had the right to be there.

Rose was up early to get ready for the day ahead. She dressed in blue slacks and a crisp white button-down shirt and wore a simple straw sun hat with a matching blue ribbon to keep the sun from her eyes. She almost looked excited. Maureen put on jeans, a short-sleeved cotton shirt and comfy shoes to accommodate the running around she expected.

The day did not disappoint. The estate sale had been advertised well, and people started showing up as soon as the items were being set out. Each had already been priced, and the agency took care of all of the sales. Maureen greeted people as they arrived and helped as she could. It was Rose, however, that made the day. She told stories of each piece of furniture and art. She let them know where they were from and how they came to fit into the house. She had stories that Maureen had never heard, and she wondered if they were all really true. Rose told stories from a safari in Africa as one couple looked at a statue that once sat in the den, and of a trip to Paris as another looked at a small painting of flowers. "We'll always have Paris," she said to no one in particular.

The enchantment she created with her stories was mesmerizing. Customers stayed longer than expected, and took home more than they had anticipated, wanting a piece of her memory. Rose was in her glory. She was the center of attention. She loved seeing people ooh and ahh over her once-loved treasures and was happy to see they would be loved by another family. There was only one time that Rose faltered: when a copy of Casablanca was found in a stack of old DVDs. Rose picked it up and held it to her chest. Maureen, knowing the meaning behind the movie, gently took it from her and put in in her purse to take home. A flicker of sadness moved across her eyes and quickly disappeared as Maureen put the movie aside. "Dad will always be with us," Maureen whispered as she put her arm around Rose's shoulder. *"On that, you can rely,"* she sang from *As Time Goes By*, knowing her mom was hearing that song in her mind. Rose smiled up at her.

The day was a success, and most things were sold by early afternoon. They retrieved a few more things throughout the day that Rose decided she couldn't part with yet, including a book of poems Grant had bought when they were dating, a scarf from Portugal, and a heart-shaped rock Rose found in the drawer of a nightstand. It was a mystery as to why she wanted a rock or why she even had it, but it was small, and she held it with such affection that Maureen couldn't take it away even if she wanted.

Rose turned over the smooth stone in her hand. It was the size of a half dollar, white with stripes of gray in it. It wasn't a perfect heart, but the shape was unmistakable. Rose remembered when she and Grant had found it. It had been tucked into the nightstand for so long that she had forgotten it was there. They were on their honeymoon in Tahoe. They had a cabin in the mountains and had spent their days hiking among the woods, picnicking by the streams and laughing. They built fires in the rock fireplace at night and shared wine on the porch under the stars.

It was the second day of the trip when Grant fell off a log into the cold stream. He screamed from the shock of the ice-cold water but came up with this treasure. He pretended he had seen it all along, but Rose knew better. She didn't care. She had kept that special stone all these years to hold the memory near and dear to her. It had been tucked away for so long. Rose smiled and giggled at the memory and knew just where she would keep it in her new place. For now, she put it in her purse, zipped up to be sure she didn't lose it.

❧

Grant met them at the hotel late in the afternoon with a notary to sign papers for the sale of the house. He could have done it for her but thought she should sign them since she was in town. The new owners were taking possession of the house when escrow closed in a week. The finality of the house being sold was hard on Rose. A few tears slowly rolled down her face as she signed the last page, signifying that a piece of her life was now over.

That night, Rose's old neighbors threw her a party to say goodbye. They had music, food, and refreshments and told stories of Rose, Grant, and the kids as they grew up. Rose had shaken off the sadness from earlier in the day. She dressed in a bright flowered dress and low pink heels. She had her hair tucked back from her face with jeweled hairpins—her go-to if a hat weren't appropriate. She laughed and spent time with each guest as they arrived.

Maureen sat back in a soft chair tucked in the corner of the living room. She listened to the sound of the voices and laughter, taking in the aroma of many family-favorite foods brought by the neighbors. Watching her mother in the crowd was surreal in a way; like watching an old family movie. It was a wonderful way to end the weekend.

There was a finality in closing the house and saying goodbye to the neighbors. Rose had a new life starting in Washington. Maureen wondered how long it would be before they would start to look for a place for Rose to be on her own. They had a pleasant routine in the house with Rose, but Maureen was sure Steve would miss their quiet time soon enough. She also knew that as soon as Rose moved out, Josh would be asking to take over the little apartment. Maureen smiled at the thought. Grace would be going away to college soon, and although they had been looking forward to more alone time, Maureen wasn't quite ready to have Josh gone too.

As she lay in bed at the hotel, her mind wandered back to the day's events. It was not just her mother saying goodbye; she too had to say goodbye to the home she grew up in and the many memories it held. Maureen rolled onto her side and looked at Rose in the next bed, who was sound asleep. There were times her mom appeared as strong and bold as a lion, but there were also times she looked small and fragile—like now. Her mother was a mystery. Maureen fell asleep reliving her mother tell the story of a trip to Africa to the family from the estate sale earlier in the day... a safari maybe?

Lions, tigers, and bears oh my.

Chapter Five

LAX always made Maureen nervous. People were everywhere, moving quickly and invading each other's space. It was like the rush hour traffic on the streets had followed them inside. They moved quickly with no regard for the people around them. She and Rose had been bumped, pushed and rushed along as passengers hurriedly made their way to their gate. After what seemed like an eternity, they finally made it to the Southwest waiting area. Exhausted in every sense of the word, she sank down in her seat, ready to fly home to Seattle.

The past two days had flown by with the final details of closing a home her parents had lived in for over 50 years. Maureen couldn't believe the number of things Mom saved over the years: everything from bottles of cough syrup that had long since expired to stacks of LIFE magazines featuring stars like Marilyn Monroe, Jackie O and The Beatles. The magazines were probably collector items, but all Maureen could think of was getting back home. She had already missed so many days at work that her vacation and sick time were nearly gone. God forbid she ever *really* got sick.

For once, Grant's business focus was a blessing—he had all the papers for the sale of the house ready. He tried to rush Mom through the process, but she asked so many questions, worried that Dad wouldn't approve. "Dad is gone—he doesn't care about the details of the sale," we kept telling her. She wanted to know all the financial details and was worried she was going to be broke. Silent tears rolled down her cheeks as she signed on the dotted line.

With a sigh, Maureen sank deeper into the hard airport seat and reached out to squeeze Mom's hand. She was happy Rose was sitting next to her with a smile on her lips. She was happily engaged in people watching; one of her favorite pastimes for as long as Maureen could remember. She closed her eyes for a minute as she took in the sweetness of the moment.

Maureen's rest was interrupted by a series of chimes. Texts were blowing up her phone, and she was thrilled—she had been waiting all day for them. Grace was out shopping with her friends for prom, and she promised to send pics of her favorite dresses. Of course, she waited until the end of the day to send them. She opened the first and saw Grace in a coral, off the shoulder, full-length dress that emphasized her dancer physique. Next was a fitted, red, backless number. She chuckled to herself as she pictured Steve having a heart attack after seeing his 18-year-old daughter in a dress so revealing. It made her smile. Rose leaned over Maureen to see what she was looking at and shouted, "With the right hairstyle, she could look just like Maureen O'Hara! She'll turn some heads for sure."

"Mom, I am right here, keep your voice down. People are looking at you." Rose looked around and smiled at anyone looking her way. She seemed to love it.

Grace kept sending more pictures, and Maureen got lost in the moment. Grace looked stunning, and she smiled at the thought of her last child going to prom. Deep in thought, she almost jumped out of her seat as an announcement boomed through the loudspeakers. "Attention all passengers on flight 363: we will begin the boarding process in ten minutes." Rose had gone to the restroom, and Maureen was getting nervous as the minutes ticked by and her mom hadn't come back. *I hope she hasn't started a conversation with another stranger. We have to board soon*, she thought. Rose had always liked to meet new people and could be found chatting with anyone, anywhere. Her habit of talking to strangers had embarrassed Maureen on more than one occasion through the years.

Thankfully, Maureen turned around and saw a young flight attendant walking with Rose toward her. Mom was chattering away, and the man was politely nodding along with the conversation. They were laughing as they drew near, and Maureen heard her mother thank the young man for walking her back to the gate.

"Your mom was turned around and couldn't remember which gate she was at, so I wanted to escort her back to you."

Maureen thanked the steward and was glad that mom made it back to them before they called them to board.

✒

As she plopped down in the gate area, Carla was instantly aware of how drained she was. She had spent the day coaching a family of ten through the dementia of the matriarch of the family. It is hard enough when it is Mom, but when she guides the family through everything and does all the cooking as well, there are a lot of layers to understand, and emotions run high. She was ready for a restful flight and time at home. She lived in the mountains outside of Seattle with her husband, and she couldn't wait to be sitting on her deck with the wind gently blowing through the trees on a starry night with a glass of deep red wine. *Just a few more hours,* she told herself.

Carla looked around the gate area at the crowd settling in to wait for the flight. There were the usual well-dressed business professionals with laptops open and phones to their ears, reviewing the day's events with colleagues. They always talked as if they were the only people in the airport, and what they had to say was critical to everyone in earshot. It made Carla chuckle. There were young couples and families going on vacation to see the space needle and pikes market. She also spotted a few military men in their fatigues, waiting together and telling stories over a beer at the nearby bar.

As Carla continued to look around, she noticed a well-dressed elderly woman. She stood out from the crowd with her unique sense of style and an exquisite hat. Carla hadn't seen hats like that in real life—just in movies or fashion magazines. It was a showpiece. The hat was deep violet, matching the floral dress she wore. Though the dress was simple in style (except for a flare at the hem), the hat was... an art piece. The deep violet linen brim dipped low on one side and had a small bouquet of wild flowers and a small butterfly set into it. She wore it with her head held high, and she smiled with ease at everyone around her. Curious, Carla watched her as the woman left her seat. The woman she was sitting with barely seemed to notice, busy with life on her phone.

Carla watched as the woman weaved in and out of the crowd, moving toward the food court. She entered the bar area, said something to the military men that made them laugh and then floated on out again into the stream of people. She was like a pinball, bouncing from one person or place to another. Carla watched until she disappeared around a corner. *I hope she gets back alright.*

Carla looked back at the younger woman, who she had overheard was her daughter. They looked alike in many ways. They shared the same build; slender with long legs, although neither seemed tall. Their light hair was neat at chin length, and both had light eyes. The only difference was the daughter's outfit: she dressed practically, wearing a collared, button-up shirt tucked into jeans and boots. As a matter of fact, she was dressed much like Carla. She looked tired, but whatever she was looking at made her smile—the same smile her mom shared so freely. Carla imagined they had the same laugh.

Carla realized she had been staring and looked away in time to see the elderly woman. Once again, she was smiling and moving through the crowd with no clear sense of direction. Carla watched as she bumped into a flight attendant at another gate. He listened to her intently, then gently took her arm and chatted with her as he escorted her back. Something about the woman was all too familiar to Carla, and she wondered about their story as the boarding call came over the loudspeaker.

The flight was going to be full. Carla took her favorite seat near the window and watched as the line rolled in behind her. Carla looked up and watched the elderly woman enter the cabin, and for a moment their eyes met. She must have taken it as a sign, as she made a beeline for the seats open next to Carla as if greeting an old friend.

She settled into the middle seat with her daughter in tow, ready for an adventure. Carla introduced herself and complimented the woman—who she now knows by Rose— on her stunning hat. That was all the incentive Rose needed to open the gates and tell Carla all about the fashion of hats. Her daughter, Maureen tried to apologize to Carla until she saw her smile and nod that it was fine. Carla asked a few questions until she saw that Rose was wearing out, and then let her fall asleep. Once she was sleeping soundly, Maureen thanked Carla for being so kind to her mom. She explained what they had been going through the last few weeks and how much she appreciated allowing her mom to rattle on.

It was then that Maureen's world was rocked—and not rocked like the "you rocked my world" type of rocked, but more like a 7.2 earthquake rocks a city and takes it to its knees. The question was simple enough. She heard it clearly, but it seemed to reverberate in her ears over and over.

"I'm wondering how long ago your mom was diagnosed with dementia?"

Maureen felt the words sting as she stared into the distance. Everything around her went still and quiet. *I am a nurse... why, why would this woman ask me that? Why would she believe that? When... How... What...* The questions assaulted her. Silenced her, in fact. She sat still for several minutes, hoping the world would stop spinning. Suddenly, she had several flashbacks of small events over the last few weeks. The house not being kept as neat as usual; pearls hidden in the silverware drawer; Mom's famous Casablanca line at the funeral causing eyes to roll; the multiple calls to 911 afterwards, leading to the hurried move; the dishwasher; forever forgetting her purse, and getting "turned around" in the neighborhood. Even the most recent red flag hadn't caught her attention: having to be escorted back to the gate by the steward.

How did I miss all the signs?

Carla saw the look in Maureen's eyes when she asked the question and realized too late that this bright woman had no idea her mom had classic signs of dementia. Carla had seen it before, and she winced at the thought. She could see how it might have happened. Rose was bigger than life; her attire spoke to a flair that few had, and it didn't seem new or unusual to Maureen. Maureen mentioned the recent loss of her dad, Grant Sr., who was a prominent doctor. It's possible—no, probable—that together in their routine her mishaps were part of her charm.

On the other hand, her husband could have been in a position where he didn't want to worry the children, so he hid his concerns—as is so often the case with couples. The spouse passes away, and only then does the family realize anything had been wrong. Carla had spent many hours coaching families through this crisis. She took a deep cleansing breath to get herself focused. Carla reached for Maureen's hand, gently squeezing it and waiting for her to respond.

The touch slowly brought Maureen back to reality. She felt the seat beneath her, and the pressure from the seat belt pulled tight against her hips. The warmth from Carla's hand on hers comforted her. She looked Carla in the eyes and was greeted by warmth and understanding. Carla was letting her take the lead when she was ready, and Maureen was grateful. It wasn't until that moment Maureen realized she had been holding her breath. She let it out slowly, then took another deep breath to calm her nerves.

"I think I need a drink," were her first words. Both women laughed, breaking the tension while Maureen wiped a tear that was starting to fall down her cheek. They called the stewardess for two red wines. Whiskey would have done the trick faster, but Maureen had questions and wanted to be able to remember the answers later. The wine was quickly delivered, and they settled into a quiet conversation.

Carla reassured Maureen that her mom appeared to be in an early stage, and it was often missed by families—especially when they live far apart, and the death of her dad made things even more cloudy. She first recommended that Maureen get Rose in to see a neurologist to get a baseline and review her medications. Maureen knew just who she wanted her mom to see. If there was ever a benefit in being a nurse, this was one of them.

Carla started with three principles to help Maureen see her mom in a different light, and therefore be able to relate to her better.

"I know your mom, who you love, is driving you a bit crazy right now," Carla started. "It may seem she is doing things on purpose. I assure you, she is not. Each day she is doing the best she can with what she has that day. Some days are good, and some are not. She doesn't know what is happening either, and that is frightening for her. Think about a time when you left the house and couldn't remember if you turned off the stove or the curling iron. You probably felt panic all through your body. Your heart raced, you felt jumpy, and you needed to know everything was alright before you could think about anything else. You probably turned the car around or called someone to go check. Even after you knew everything was fine, you still found your heart racing a bit." Maureen certainly knew that feeling and nodded in understanding.

"For someone with dementia, they get that same feeling of panic but can't relate it to a specific item. It's a general feeling, like a panic attack. There isn't any way to check to know things are OK. All they know is something isn't right." Maureen's face scrunched up, and her brows were knit together as she thought about what this must feel like. She looked down at her mom and wondered how often she might have felt like that since dad had passed.

"What do I do?"

"Give her grace. Believe she is doing the best she can with what she is given that day. Slow down; your mom is bright and full of life, but information takes longer to process. If she feels she has time to respond, it will help her relax. I once had a gentleman I was coaching who told me he would ask his wife a question like, 'Do you want ham or chicken on your sandwich?' She didn't respond, so he went into the kitchen and started lunch. Minutes later she came in and said 'chicken.' He barely remembered the question, and she might not have either, but she was happy as could be." Carla paused to see if Maureen was understanding. They ordered a second glass of wine, and she continued on.

"Next, realize that we are all trying to make sense of our world. So, to do that, we are sometimes inventive. We connect truths, connecting the dots in a way, although they may have little basis in fact. Remember the pearls that you found in the kitchen drawer at your moms? How did she explain them being there?"

Maureen thought about that morning. It was busy. They were getting ready for a full day starting with the funeral service, burial and a long reception afterwards. There would be hundreds of people there, and they were already exhausted. Maureen began to tell Carla the events of that day. "Mom wanted to wear her pearls with her black dress, but she couldn't find them anywhere. They had looked all through the house to no avail. I had given up and went to get coffee and a quick bite to eat. When I went to grab a knife from the drawer, something at the back drew my attention, and I saw the pearls tucked inside a plastic bag. It struck me as strange at the time. Mom is always so particular with her jewelry. I showed Mom where I found the pearls and asked her why she put them there. Mom said that the housekeeper must have hidden them there. 'She was up to no good,' she joked. I was too preoccupied to figure out my mother's crazy story at the time, but I figured I would talk to the housekeeper later in the week."

Carla chimed in with a simple, yet important observation. "You see, there are two truths there. Rose has a pearl necklace, and it was not in its place in her jewelry box. How it got in the silverware drawer is the story or bridge she created for it to make sense. It wouldn't make sense for her to do it herself—that would be ridiculous. Pearls go in their bag in the jewelry box; that is where she always put them. So, her mind creates a story that makes sense to her. It bridges the two truths. We all fill in the blanks in our lives. With dementia, the truths are farther apart, and the bridge is connected to the emotion felt at the time."

"Thank you, Carla. It is beginning to make sense now."

Carla broke the seriousness by commenting on the resemblance between Maureen and Rose that she had noticed in the airport. Sitting close and getting to know Maureen, it was even more obvious.

"Have you ever looked in the mirror and thought, 'Oh my God, when did my mother get here?'" Maureen laughed, remembering the feeling every morning when she first looked in the mirror.

"We all feel that way," Carla smiled knowingly. "In our mind, we are still that youthful person inside of us, and then the mirror tells us differently. We look at pictures of ourselves and wonder who replaced our face and body. We remember how we felt at an event and the picture doesn't match the memory. I do NOT like pictures. They make me look… my age." Carla laughed, and Maureen joined her as they lamented their beauty woes.

"If we all do this, what does it have to do with dementia?" Maureen asked.

"In those with dementia, the picture gets stuck at certain age ranges. The most common is 30's to 40's, when their children were young and their careers were flourishing. These time periods have strong emotions tied to them. At times, those with dementia will talk about someone from their past or tell stories from long ago as if were happening now. The memory is *that* strong. My own grandfather called me by my mom's name all the time in conversations. I would ignore the reference and continue the conversation. As he would chat with me, he would realize I wasn't my mom and acknowledge me as me. I didn't make a big deal of it, and he was relaxed, so his memories were able to float up. It didn't always work, but it did enough to make it worthwhile.

"If you listen to someone speak, it will tell you where they are in their memories. If they talk about work or babies in the present tense, it gives you a hint of where they are in memories. Knowing a lot about time periods in your mom's life will help you when she mentions someone you have never heard of. Remember, your mom, like all of us, had a life before her children came along. Having met your mom for a short time, I bet she has some stories tucked in her memory that will surprise you. Learning them will be a gift."

Carla liked Maureen. She reminded her of herself, struggling with her own mom's diagnosis years before. Like Carla, Maureen had children, a new grandbaby, a career, and a husband who adored her. These would be tested over time, and Carla knew the family had a long road ahead of them. Carla felt connected to Maureen.

The captain's voice broke into the conversation as they were finishing their second glass of wine. "Good evening folks, we're moving into our final stretch and will be starting our descent into Seattle momentarily. Please make sure your seatbelts are securely fastened, and your tray tables and seats are in their upright and locked positions." It was time to land already. Carla should have been exhausted, but instead, she felt accomplished and energized. She reached into her bag and gave Maureen her card. "Please call me at the first of the week. I want to know how things are going and see if we can plan to meet up again."

Rose woke up when the seat backs had to be raised. She fixed her hair, placed her hat smartly on her head, and touched up her makeup. She really was a stunning woman. She carried on a conversation about the family. She was proud of Maureen and her career. She bragged about her and her grandchildren. She asked if Carla had seen the prom gowns. The last few minutes of the flight were all about how stunning Grace looked. "Much like my younger years!" she exclaimed. She talked about jewelry and hairstyles and even suggested a hat to top it all off.

The three gathered their luggage, hugged, and said good-bye. Carla watched as they walked away toward Steve in his waiting car. Rose was dancing among the crowd, flashing her smile, and those she connected with smiled instantly. She was a true joy to be around—something dementia had not yet stolen.

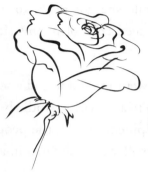

Chapter Six

aureen had a lot on her mind after the revelation she received on the plane ride home that her mom—bright and beautiful as she was—probably had dementia. It was like looking back after finishing a mystery novel and suddenly recognizing all the pieces that pointed to the culprit.

She had a couple of days to process and talk to Steve about the possibility before she would see Carla again. Carla was going to be a guest on the television show *Home and Family in the Pacific Northwest* and had invited Maureen to sit in the audience and have coffee afterwards.

In just the past few days, Maureen had called a neurologist she knew, Dr. Karen Brad, and made an appointment for Rose to be seen the following week. It gave her a sense of control over the situation. It felt better to take action, even if it were only setting an appointment. She desperately needed to do something.

Maureen grinned. "Nurses like control," she said to herself under her breath while she got ready to go to the television studio. "I clearly need control in this situation," she said, and sighed.

She drove to the studio, went in, and found a seat in the audience. She had never been to a television studio before and was fascinated with the equipment and all the people managing the set. It was much smaller than she had imagined.

"Good morning, and welcome to *Home and Family in the Pacific Northwest!*" the hosts, Terri and Mark began with a Hollywood smile. "Today we have some special guests coming your way."

The show began with a cooking demo from a local chef. The food smelled wonderful, even from the demo alone— Italian sausage with pasta in a spicy red sauce. Maureen's stomach took notice and growled. She popped a hard candy in her mouth in an attempt to curb her hunger. Carla was scheduled next, and she was anxious to hear her speak.

Mark and Terri were both young and good looking. *Aren't they always?* Maureen thought as the host began the introduction for Carla.

Mark's deep voice interrupted her train of thought, and she turned her attention back to the stage. "These days, balancing a family has a lot more pressures than just work, home life, taking the kids to school and extracurricular activities. Our next guest is going to help us understand the demands on parents when they must balance life between their children and their aging parents. Please help me welcome Carla Veloza to the stage."

The studio erupted in applause as Carla entered the stage smiling at the audience, both on the set and on camera. She looked relaxed and confident. This was the first time Maureen had seen Carla since the flight, and she was too emotional on the plane to take notice of Carla's appearance. She could hear her voice, smooth and calm in her ears, but her looks were a bit of a blur.

Maureen watched her as she came in and took her seat. Carla was slightly shorter than she was, maybe 5' 2" at most, but she walked tall. Today she was dressed in a tailored black skirt and short jacket. An emerald green blouse tucked neatly in the skirt softly billowed in the front, softening the overall look. She looked fit and healthy, like someone who worked out regularly but enjoyed the outdoors as well. She wore light makeup, and her jewelry was simple.

Maureen would have pegged her as a no-nonsense type until you saw her smile which showed all the way to her eyes. *I remember those eyes*, Maureen thought. They were green with gold flecks; warm and reassuring.

"Welcome, Carla. We would love to get to know a bit about you and how you got started working with the elderly," Terri's cheerful voice interrupted Maureen's thoughts yet again.

"Thank you. I am happy to share my story with you and your audience," Carla said as she looked at the crowd and then back to the host.

"I had been a counselor, school psychologist, and sales manager before I found my calling with seniors in the early 90's. It came very naturally to me. I grew up with my maternal grandparents in my home. They moved in when I was two years old, and were still there after I left on my own."

Maureen took a quick breath, realizing how much Carla's story was similar to her own. She leaned forward in her seat, intent on hearing every word Carla had to say.

"My grandmother—my father's only parent—passed away while I was pregnant with my daughter, Twila. She never met the grandparent who I had spent so many summers living with learning to sew." A soft smile crossed Carla's face. "A year later, my grandfather Poppy, who had lived with me since I was a toddler, passed away. Then, a couple of years later, the day my son Christian was born, my grandmother, Vovo, died after a difficult hospital stay. She was the last of that generation. I couldn't travel at the time, so I didn't get to say goodbye to her."

Carla paused and took a slow breath, continuing on. "A day shy of one month later, I was offered a job in a nursing home as the Social Services Director, and I took it as a gift back to my grandparents." Carla took another slow breath, letting the story sink in. "After 26 years, it is *still* a gift I could never repay."

Terri and Mark both took a deep breath as Terri wiped a tear from her eye. "That is a touching story. Thank you for sharing it," Mark said softly and smiled.

Terri then started on the topic at hand. "I understand that there is a term called the 'Sandwich Generation,' describing how families have to balance their life. I wonder if the audience knows just what the Sandwich Generation is. Can you give them a brief description?"

"Yes of course," Carla replied. "The term Sandwich Generation was coined in 1981 to describe adults in their 30's to 40's raising children *and* caring for their parents. Today it has shifted to those in their 40's to 60's whose children are 18 years or older, yet still need support, and their parents whose needs are ever changing. Children are staying home longer and are moving back home after college and life events, like losing a job, divorce, or trying to save to buy a first home. An astounding 47% of adults today fall into this stage of life."

"My own children, now grown, still need me for emotional support, life advice, and occasional financial support." The audience let out an understanding laugh. "At the same time, my mom needs me to follow her medical care and be her voice and memory with doctors. I worry about her just like I worried about my children when they were growing up. I *am* an adult in the Sandwich Generation, caught between supporting my children and my parents."

There it was again, Maureen thought. *My story in her life.*

"What does this mean for those in the Sandwich Generation? How does it affect their life?" Mark asked.

Carla continued with the same wise, compassionate voice Maureen remembered from the plane. "For some, taking care of their parents turns into a full-time job. Most of their time is spent dealing with medical issues—medications and doctors' visits, cooking meals and paying bills, and the most feared—the loss of independence or memory loss. This might mean hands-on care for part or all of the day, as well as the night. On the other hand, many are trying to balance their families and careers with the long-distance understanding and navigation of their parent's needs."

Terri pressed on, "What advice would you give people living in the Sandwich Generation?"

Carla answered without hesitation, "After working over 26 years in the senior industry, I would offer one piece of advice: take care of *yourself*," she paused. "I have seen it time and time again—a selfless family member taking wonderful care of their loved one ends up in the hospital because they neglected their own medical, social, physical, and spiritual needs. They forgot the essential understanding that taking care of themselves *allows* them to take care of the one they love. They left the balance behind in trying to care for their parents."

"Can you give us, say, five life balancing ideas for our audience to start with?" Mark chimed in again, not skipping a beat.

Carla faced more of the audience as she spoke this time. "Let's turn our attention to the screen as we move through the top five life-balancing ideas I recommend." As the first slide went up, Maureen found herself thankful to have these tips in writing. They were both practical and incredibly relevant to her life.

1. **Finding support**: this may be a spouse, sibling, a local support group or a friend. Anyone who will let you laugh, cry, and let it all out. A shoulder to lean on. Someone who will bring you coffee, make you dinner, take you out, and pay close attention to your needs along the way. A person who will be honest and tell you when you need a break, and will then help you make it happen.

2. **Taking breaks and doing something for yourself each day**: this could be something as small as a walk outside to smell the fresh air. Little things like this can do wonders when your mind is racing with work and worry. For me, taking a walk in nature, drawing up a hot, relaxing bath, or watching a favorite television show gives me an escape.

3.   **The power of breathing**: take a deep breath with your eyes closed, and repeat a few times. While you exhale, let go of all thoughts of the world around you; let them fade away. Picture yourself wrapped in your favorite color, and feel it comforting you. As you breathe slowly in and out, take notice of how your body relaxes. When you practice deep breathing on a regular basis, you can get back to this relaxed state with just one breath. Your body will remember how you felt, and your deep breath will remind it to relax. This is my go-to throughout any busy day.

4.   **Be healthy**: be mindful of what you are eating and make sure you are getting enough sleep. The brain heals when you sleep, and it helps sort out the problems of the day giving you fresh ideas and strength in the morning.

5.   **Be realistic**: ask for help when you need it, hire a professional to help with small things, and listen to advice and insight from others. Reaching out is a sign of strength.

"*You* are not alone. Remember, there are 47% of adults your age in the same stage of life—band together and support one another. You are in good company."

"Any last thoughts?" Terri asked.

Carla paused one last time, then spoke earnestly. "There will always be a Sandwich Generation; our children and parents will still be around and will need us in various ways throughout our lives. Be strong, be balanced, and laugh whenever you can."

"Thank you, Carla..." Mark's voice trailed away as music began to play. The audience clapped loudly as the show went on to a commercial break, and Carla disappeared backstage. Maureen sat back in her seat, replaying the show in her mind. She was glad she had it recording on her DVR at home so she could catch anything she might have missed.

The show continued with a local musician and ended with a segment on a Pinterest-style kitchen herb garden for the herbs that the chef had used in the cooking demo at the start of the show.

Maureen stayed glued to her seat as prizes were announced to the audience for coming. All of the *Home and Family* guests, for the most part, came out to do a round of questions and answers. Maureen saw Carla as she came from behind the curtain to address the audience. There were a lot of questions, but Maureen didn't care. Maybe someone would ask a question she hadn't thought of previously.

Carla sat on a high stool in front of the audience, smiling as she turned her attention back to the crowd. "Does anyone have a question?"

"How do I know when my parents need help? They always say they are fine," a woman sitting near Maureen called out.

"That is the most common question I get asked. Do they live near you?" The woman nodded yes.

Carla continued, "It should start with a good look around when you visit your parents. Is a normally clean, neat house looking more 'lived in' when you come over? Does the food in the fridge look fresh? Do you get one of those 'huh' kind of feelings, like something is not quite right?" Carla looked at the woman for an acknowledgement that she understood. The woman was nodding, so Carla went on.

"If you are able, look at medication bottles and see if the prescription makes sense. If the prescription is dated over a month ago, but the bottle is still half full, or there is more than one type of pill in the same bottle, you might have a problem."

Another hand shot up, bursting out with a question before Carla could even call on him. "How do you figure it all out?! They confuse *me*," an older man asked, maybe for himself.

"If it is your medication—or your parents' and they are cooperative—take all the medications in the house they are using, including all over the counter medications, to their pharmacy and ask for help. You're right. It is complicated, but the pharmacist is there to help you. They will tell you if something seems off. They will also show you drug interactions and which over the counter medications may interfere with the ones prescribed by the doctor. In this day and age, we have so many different specialists that there may even be prescriptions that are blocking the effects of another without knowing it. Furthermore, you will get information from the pharmacist about how each medication is to be taken. Then, when you have the information, you can make decisions on how to best be sure that they are taken at the right time, in the right dose, and by the right method."

"I have time for one more question…" Carla announced as she looked over the audience. "Yes, your question?" Carla asked a woman who looked distraught with her hand barely held high enough to see.

"My mom, she seems to be fine physically, but she is so negative. Everything I—or anyone, for that matter—does is wrong in her eyes… and she hoards. She has books, magazines, and newspapers everywhere. I can't even see the floor in her home. She won't let me get rid of anything. She used to collect things, but now… now it is just so bad, and it seems only to be getting worse." The women spoke softly at first, getting louder as she finally let it all out.

Carla paused, wanting to choose her words carefully. "There are many reasons a person holds on to things, even seemingly insignificant things. It could be something that has always been there. Now that she doesn't have other things like work or family to keep her occupied, the hoarding is out of control. She is symbolically holding on to something, or someone. I like to say that 'as a person ages, they become more of themselves. It's much like a sauce that reduces, and the flavors become more intense.' That said, the hoarding could also be as a result of a loss of some kind that she is desperately trying to hold onto, symbolically." The woman who had been listening broke down into tears. Carla left her seat and gently took her aside to talk privately.

Maureen watched from afar as Carla spoke to the woman. She could imagine the gentle tone in her voice she would be sharing advice with and knew the woman would receive her full attention. She watched as Carla gave her a card and wrote something on the back. The woman looked at it, nodded, and left.

The last *Home and Family* guest had just finished answering questions as Carla approached Maureen.

She greeted Maureen warmly, "I am so happy you were able to be here! Do you still have time to get some coffee? I would love to hear how you are doing, and hear about Rose."

"Yes, I have the day off. My mom is busy with all the things we brought home from her house, so I don't have to rush."

Maureen and Carla left the studio for their cars and met up in Bothell at a small local coffee shop. On arriving, they each ordered a latte and found some oversized chairs in a corner where they could talk.

"Thank you so much for inviting me to the show. It really hit home. I didn't realize I was part of a 'special generation.' I must admit though, I have seen it. At work, I see families trying to make decisions for their parents all the time. I never thought much about the weight of the children and family they may have at home; my attention is so focused on the patient we are trying to take care of. I sure do get it now," Maureen laughed. "I will have much more empathy in the future."

"It's easy to get caught up in what we have to accomplish. The families you work with in the future will benefit from your own revelations and new experiences," Carla reassured her.

Maureen caught Carla up on the upcoming neurologist appointment the following week. The appointment with Dr. Karen would give them a baseline on Rose's cognitive state, and if needed, they would look at medication to help her stay stable for a longer period of time. Carla was happy to hear that Maureen was acting so quickly. She understood that some families had a hard time grasping the concept of dementia in their parents and stay in denial, losing precious time in the early stages.

"There are a few things you can do to help the brain stay 'fit,' especially in these early stages," Carla said, giving some hope to Maureen. "Any activity that requires you to give all of your attention will help. Games like Sudoku or riddles require you to focus solely on them in order to find answers.

There are easy 1-4 sudoku games to start with, and you can build to 6 or 9 numbers. Honestly, I am not good at the larger number ones, but I try. Learning a new language is also a great exercise for the brain."

"How about crossword puzzles?" Maureen asked.

"Crossword puzzles are route memory tasks. For the most part, either you know the answer, or you don't, so they do not meet the *full focus* requirement. Of course, it wouldn't hurt to do them. Any activity we have to really concentrate on is a good activity," Carla went on. "Nowadays there are some great online programs that can be fun and helpful too. I bet your kids can find some and help get them set up. It will give them a role to play in an area they feel comfortable in."

Maureen nodded, already thinking of solutions. "We have an iPad that hasn't been used. I can have them download some things on it, so Mom doesn't get… uh, *creative* on the computer. She has already managed to get the remotes on the TVs to do some interesting things. Steve went out while we were gone and found a super simple remote with minimal buttons for Mom's room. So far, so good, but it *has* only been a couple days!" Maureen and Carla laughed like old friends sharing memories.

She is so easy to talk to, Maureen thought.

The two women finished their coffee, chatting about life over two pieces of buckwheat banana bread spread with fresh cinnamon cream cheese that the coffee shop had on special.

They put aside the talks about Rose and dementia to spend time getting to know one another. They had many interests that were the same, and each of them had a unique story to share.

Carla told Maureen about the time she and her husband, Clif, were hiking to Spider Meadow near Leavenworth and saw a porcupine coming down the road—all quills fully extended. "We could see the animal coming down the trail way ahead of us. A dog had run past us a few minutes prior, so we thought it was another dog at first. You could see two people coming down the trail just behind it. As we got closer, we thought, *now that is one ugly dog!*

"Then as we got closer still, we saw it was a porcupine, quills sticking straight out as he waddled in front of the hikers. We beelined it off the trail and up the side of the hill to get out of its way, but the dog that had passed us started to come back up the trail. The hikers called out to the dog, and he sat down in the middle of the trail. They stopped behind the porcupine, and it stopped as well. Then, in the blink of an eye, it drew in all its quills and dove under the brush on the side of the road. You could see the brush moving as it sped down the hill. It was watching a live cartoon!" They laughed out loud as Carla acted out the movement of the animal. "I am going to have to go there to hike; Steve would love it!" Maureen said between breaths as she laughed.

Maureen was still laughing as she told a hiking story of her own. "You don't have to be out in the wilderness to encounter a wild animal. Steve and I love to walk the trail through McWhirter Park in Redmond. We had finished our loop and were heading back through a small path that borders the park on one side and the horse ranches on the other side. We stopped on a small high bridge over the river to catch our breath and check out the stream, when I saw what looked like a large dark brown dog downstream from us walking our way. I pointed it out to Steve, and he took a double take. It was not a dog; it was a bear cub! Not knowing where the mother bear was, we got out of there, *FAST.* We forgot all the rules of not turning your back on a bear and staying calm. We ran! I am sure the bear cub didn't even know we were there, but our hearts were racing. We have never seen another one there, but we pay waaaay more attention when we walk now." Again, both women laughed, enjoying the ease of the conversation.

A few hours had passed before either had realized it. It was the most relaxing afternoon Maureen had had since her father had passed months before. Carla agreed that it was refreshing for her as well. She had been busy for the past few weeks and would be leaving for another trip the following Monday.

They walked out to their cars and said goodbye, scheduling lunch (with Rose this time) in about a month. Both would have enjoyed it sooner, but schedules were not having it.

֍

Carla replayed the day that evening as she sat on her porch under the stars. This was the spot she and Clif loved to sit and relax in the evening. They would often enjoy a glass of wine and relax after the sun went down. On a cool night, like tonight, they lit the outdoor heater and listened to the breeze through the trees on the property. The dogs lay at their feet and music played on the Echo.

Carla thought about the television show in the morning and how she was able to share her own story as part of the education on the Sandwich Generation. She was thankful for the opportunity to not only share with the audience that morning but connect with Maureen over coffee—who, to her surprise, was so much like herself.

It always touched Carla's heart to tell the story of her family. There were so many different stories she could share between a grandmother who was the youngest of 18—there were 16 girls and 2 boys and a grandfather who was the middle of 5 siblings. Growing up, every family gathering happened at Carla's home. There were countless parties, and they were always large. Family traditions, mostly around food and laughter, are what she remembered the most.

Her father's family was small in comparison. It was just her grandmother, Gram, and her aunt, Twila, who Carla had named her daughter after, and a few cousins. Carla spent summers with her grandmother in a small apartment for several years. There she learned to sew, cook and do embroidery.

Carla smiled at the memory of snuggling with Gram and drinking hot chocolate late at night when she couldn't sleep.

Carla was glad she wrote down her family stories years before in a journal while she was expecting. Carla understood how important sharing your history could be. There are some things only you will ever know unless you share it. Family histories have a tendency to fade away.

Getting to know people like Maureen was what Carla liked best about her career. She was able to build relationships with those she counseled. Connecting families and their history to someone who they were feeling separated from was truly a gift.

Chapter Seven

Carla sat on the deck at Duke's Seafood and Chowder on a beautiful Seattle afternoon, waiting for Maureen and Rose to arrive. It was a warm spring day, and she was taking full advantage of it. It had been just over a month since meeting Maureen for coffee after the taping of the show. Carla looked forward to seeing them both. She hadn't seen Rose since the airport and wondered if Rose would remember her.

Carla saw them as they walked down the sidewalk toward the restaurant. Maureen was dressed in light slacks and an airy blouse, and Rose wore a vibrant red cotton dress with small white flowers imprinted on it, perfectly fitting to her personality. Another unique hat sat tilted to the right on her head, dipping low over her eye. This one was white with red ribbon and netting at the wide brim. Carla smiled and admired the style that Rose pulled off so well. It all looked so natural on her.

The pair waved hello and walked closer as they recognized Carla on the deck.. Rose wore that charming smile she gave away so freely, and Carla couldn't help but smile back at her.

"It is so nice to see you again," Rose said as she took Carla's hand, sitting down at the table.

Had she actually remembered her, or did Maureen remind Rose of who she was? Carla wasn't certain, as Rose seemed so sure of herself.

"It is good to see you both as well," Carla responded as the waiter approached with menus.

They listened to the specials of the day and perused the menus for a few minutes, chit-chatting about the weather. The restaurant had music playing overhead, and Rose knew the words to almost every song. She sang along, maybe a bit too loud. Maureen worried that she was bothering the other tables, but no one seemed to notice her. Rose swayed to the music as she sang, almost dancing in her seat.

Maureen, feeling a bit embarrassed by her mom, felt the need to give Carla some insight into her behavior. "My mom and dad loved music. They went dancing all the time. They even brought home a dance trophy from a country club dance! Sometimes, when Grant and I were young, we would see them dancing in the kitchen by candlelight. I would sit on top of the stairs and watch them spin under the dim light. It is one of my favorite memories of the two of them."

"You were supposed to be sleeping," Rose chided her. They all laughed at Rose's scolding.

"Music is powerful," Carla shared. "Songs that have importance to us or are connected to strong memories wake up the whole brain. You don't just hear the music; you sense the memory in sight and touch too. You might even remember a scent from a song."

"What was your and Grant's song?" Carla asked.

In unison, Maureen and Rose sang "As Time Goes By" from the movie *Casablanca*.

"Well, no question there! I bet you have some magical memories related to that song," Carla encouraged Rose.

Rose blushed as she shared her and Grant's love of the classic movie *Casablanca* and how whenever that song came on, they danced—even during the movie. They had watched it on their first date and had seen it over 50 times since then. The song and movie were their anthem. Maureen nodded in agreement, turning to look at her mom. She knew Rose's heart still broke about Dad's passing. *No matter what the future brings.... As time goes by...* Maureen continued the lyric in her mind.

The waiter brought them all back down to reality when he returned to get their orders. He answered a couple questions on the menu before they all ordered chowder in bread bowls and a calamari appetizer to share.

As they waited for their meals, Carla turned to Rose.

"How do you like Seattle?"

"Oh, I love being here with Maureen and the family. Did Maureen tell you about the lovely room Steve created for me? It is delightful. He painted it in my favorite colors and built the most unique area to store my hats. It is a work of art. I can be close to everyone but still have some quiet space. You know, having all the young ones around—I guess not sooo young," she murmured, "can be… quite noisy and busy. I love them, but sometimes I need to rest," Rose was excited, and everything spilled out in what seemed like one big breath.

Carla was about to respond, but in the next breath, Rose continued. It was softer and slower this time, "You know, I've had some trouble since my Grant—my husband— passed away. I guess my memory isn't what it used to be," she sighed.

"It's definitely been hard since Grant passed," Carla echoed.

"Yes, I miss him. We were so good together. Like Bogart and Bergman," Rose had a faraway look in her eyes as she spoke. *Casablanca... it truly was their movie*, Carla thought as she watched her.

The waiter approached the table with their meals, and Rose greeted him with a smile and light conversation as he served the calamari and chowders as if she had never mentioned Grant. Carla and Maureen let the moment pass without bringing it back up.

Maureen and Carla spent some time catching up on life as they ate, sharing stories of hiking and home. Life was busy for Maureen; prom was just a couple weeks away, and graduation would soon follow. Carla had been on the road with seminars and had another set starting soon, but this time they would be held in England. Clif would be joining her for a week afterwards to travel around and enjoy being tourists. The conversation moved along easily, just as it had the last time.

Carla wanted to ask about the doctor's appointment Rose would have had by now but wanted to let Maureen set the pace on the conversation about Rose. They were about halfway through lunch when Maureen stepped into that conversation.

"We went to the doctors a few weeks ago," she began, nodding towards Rose. "Dr. Karen was thorough. She ran blood tests, scans, and memory testing."

"It took forever for them to figure out my memory isn't what it used to be," Rose chimed in. "I could have told them that!"

Maureen glanced at Rose, rolled her eyes, and continued, "The medical tests came out pretty well, but the memory test…" Maureen was having trouble remembering the name of the test. It amazed her that even as a nurse, she was having a hard time with all the information she was receiving on dementia. *It's different when it's your own mom,* she realized internally.

"The MMSE, Mini-Mental State Exam?" Carla asked.

"Yes, that was it. Mom scored a 21 out of 30. The doctor thought Mom did pretty well," Maureen replied, looking for confirmation.

"She did," Carla agreed, smiling at Rose.

"I missed a few things," Rose admitted. "But, I was able to spell the word *world* backwards… D.L.R.O.W. Bet that surprised them!" she grinned at the thought. It hadn't surprised Maureen though, as her mother was amazing at spelling—a talent Maureen hadn't inherited. She went by the belief, "Spelling is inversely related to intelligence." It didn't say much for her mom, but at least it made Maureen feel good.

"I bet it did," Carla said, agreeing with her and enjoying the pride that Rose had in her accomplishment.

Rose seemed to be taking the conversation about her doctor's visit in stride, so Carla explained the results to them. "The MMSE does show some memory challenges. Scores below 26 demonstrate some cognitive decline," Carla stared, looking over at Rose to see how she was handling the information. Rose looked back at her with interest, so Carla continued. "It means there is a mild cognitive impairment that may show up in any number of ways."

"Like learning how to use the remote or the dishwasher? Those things give me fits!" Rose declared.

"Exactly! Some things are easy, and at times, other things don't make much sense. It's as if the thought or knowledge is just out of reach or at the tip of your tongue, but you can't get it out," Carla was giving words to what Rose felt, and she was nodding her head in agreement.

"What else did the doctor say?" Carla asked, moving the conversation forward.

"They started her on Aricept. A low dose," Maureen added. "It is supposed to help slow the memory loss down; stabilize it."

"That is a great place to start," Carla turned her attention back to Rose. "How are you feeling with the medication?"

"A little sleepy at first, but now I feel fine. My mind feels more awake. I think it helps," Rose explained.

"Glad to hear it," Carla replied.

The waiter had come back to clear the plates and offered dessert. They split two, as it was a perfect time to indulge. The first was the Pier Pie: a chocolate and espresso ice cream layered in a cookie crust with all-natural chocolate sauce, homemade whipped cream and topped with toasted almonds. The second was the "I Want You So Bad" marionberry pie with wild Washington marionberries, served with a scoop of vanilla ice cream.

They all agreed that the second pie was really just a serving of fruit, and that made it good for them. They also agreed to take a walk around the lake after lunch to work them off. It would be worth it.

The three walked down to the lake after dessert, each complaining that they were too full, feeling like they were waddling like the ducks around the lake. They laughed as they went. Turning a corner, Rose noticed a college rowing crew on the lake.

"Oh look. The rowing crew is practicing!" Rose exclaimed and moved quickly to the rail to watch. Maureen and Rose followed. Maureen had never seen her mom take an interest in any sort of sport, so she was curious about her excitement now.

Rose watched with apt interest. "Even it out girls!" she urged them. "Ugh, she is hanging at the catch," she seemed exasperated. "Bury the blade!" Rose yelled at them. "That's it, now push for ten!" she cheered.

"Uhm, Mom? What are you doing yelling at them? Stop." Maureen was embarrassed and had no idea what language her mother was talking. "What are you yelling at them?" Was she more confused than they all thought?

"Oh, honey. They need to practice a whole lot more if they want to get anywhere in competition. When I rowed, we were magnificent," Rose beamed with pride as she stated her fact.

"Mom, you ne—" Maureen began, but Carla broke in, "Rose, tell me about your rowing crew."

Maureen looked at Carla and then back to her mom as Rose began to tell stories of her college experiences on the rowing team. She started to interrupt again, but Carla raised her hand to stop her so Rose didn't get interrupted. Carla's eyes never left Rose's face.

Rose took off with her story. "You know, rowing didn't become part of the Olympics for women until 1976, at the Montreal games, but women have had rowing crews since the early 1900's. They were mostly through colleges. We were all jealous of the men who got to qualify and compete in the Olympics. We all dreamt about it being open to women one day," she stole a glance at the lake before continuing. "Their keel—their balance—is rock solid," she looked at the ladies with pride.

"We were up early and worked hard. Did you know that is how I got my figure? You are in good shape when you're rowing for hours each morning. Worked too, I got your father's attention!" Rose was giddy while telling her stories. She struck a pose as she might have back then with her hand on her hip, tilting her head toward an imaginary camera. "I think I have a few pictures in one of those old albums at the house. I haven't done it since college, but it stays in the blood. Our crew was a sculling quad; that means four rowers, each with two oars. We called our team Eagles Wings, because we flew across the lake," Rose made a swoosh sound as she waved her hand across the air and turned to watch the crews finish their practice. Once more, she was captivated by the crew on the lake.

Maureen looked at her mom with a mixture of disbelief and astonishment, shaking her head in confusion. Rose had always been the social butterfly, prim and proper. A perfect doctor's wife, deeply engaged in society. She held garden parties and was on committees. She led volunteer projects with her church. She wore dresses and hats all the time. The thought of her being a "jock" in college was giving Maureen's mind something to reconcile. Seeing Rose now in her red dress and white hat didn't quite fit the image, and it made the thought even harder to comprehend. *What else don't I know? And how the heck did Carla get her to share this part of her life?*

Rose stayed by the rail and watched as the crew raced across the lake, occasionally cheering them on with a smile that spread across her whole face. Maureen and Carla sat on a bench nearby watching her.

"How did you know?" Maureen asked.

"I didn't," Carla said, smiling. "I just let her tell me what she was thinking. What came out was what was floating to the top of her memory. I let her share that with us without judgement or question. Once she got started, there was a lot to tell." The two women looked back at Rose, and she was glowing with excitement.

"It doesn't matter to me if the story is true, partly true, or not true at all. I just open the door and accept what comes out. Using a simple line like, 'Tell me about...' gives her the opportunity to say whatever is there," Carla explained. "I use it all the time. 'Tell me about your husband, tell me about your home, tell me about your job.' Simply fill in the blank with whatever fits the conversation."

"I would have never known *my own mother* if you hadn't interrupted me. Thank you."

Maureen thought of all the times she had stopped her mother from telling a "story" lately or had corrected her. She shuddered at the thought and wondered how much more she would know of her mother if she had listened and been open to her stories. *In five minutes, I learned about a chapter in my mom's life I didn't know existed. All it took was five minutes.* Maureen rolled the thought over and over again in her mind.

The crew came in to shore, and Rose went over to greet them. She "talked shop" with the girls about their performance on the water and had the girls laughing with her in no time. Rose wished them well as the crew packed up. She then walked over to join Carla and Maureen on the bench.

After just a few seconds, Rose stood up. "Ready?" She had energy and wanted to get moving again. Maureen and Carla stood up and stretched, and they continued their stroll around the lake. They stopped along the way to enjoy the sunshine and feed the wild—well, local anyways—ducks leftover bread from lunch, being careful not to get caught. "You aren't supposed to feed the ducks," Carla had been told once by a passerby.

As they walked, Rose told stories about Maureen and Grant as children. "We spent many days at the park. Maureen jumped in a fountain to swim and grab coins, while Grant played ball on a team for many years. We had picnics with fried chicken and watermelon spread out on checkered tablecloths, and spent a lot of time swinging." Maureen had gotten the hang of listening without correction and kept saying, "Tell me about it Mom… tell me more." And more she got. Rose told stories for the next 45 minutes. She was lively and animated.

Maureen raised her eyebrows at Carla when she didn't remember the story the same way or knew the facts weren't right, but she kept it to herself. It didn't really matter anyway. Seeing her mom filled with such life and energy was what she needed today. This was a practice Maureen was going to use for a long time.

They arrived back at Duke's having made the long loop and said goodbye. It had been an eventful afternoon, and Rose was wearing out. Her energy was well spent with all the walking and storytelling.

Carla watched them as they walked to their car and then turned around to go to her own.

⤚

Maureen appreciated the long ride home. Mom had fallen asleep within a block of the restaurant, allowing Maureen to listen to music and relax. She was singing along to a favorite from the 70's, "Make it with You" by Bread, when she realized the truth in what Carla had shared about the power of songs for herself. That song played at every dance she went to throughout high school. She remembered her high school boyfriend and how awkward he was slow dancing, not knowing where to put his hands. She could smell the popcorn served with sweet punch in the back of the gym, and she could feel the beating of their hearts. She remembered crying over the song when they broke up, and how heartbroken she was. The song really did bring her back.

Maureen suddenly understood the strength of her parents' song, "As Time Goes By." Their song had so many more memories attached to it. Maureen knew it was more than just the song. The whole movie had so much meaning for them. They knew every line by heart and had always used them in their own romantic way. It was almost like a secret language they shared. Mom still repeated many of the lines. She had used one at the funeral to say goodbye to Dad. "Kiss me, kiss me as if it were the last time." Grant thought it was eccentric, but Maureen knew it was their love language.

Maureen looked over at her mom and understood how her heart must break every time she heard the song. And still, it brought her back to her best memories... of Dad.

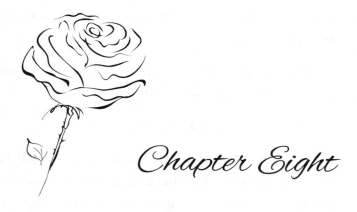

Chapter Eight

ime was moving too fast. Before she knew it, Maureen was caught in a whirlwind of activities surrounding Grace's graduation. The first item on the calendar was prom. Nowadays, getting ready for prom turned out to be a weeklong event. To start the week off, Grace and Maureen went together to pick up her gown. Grace had finally found the perfect one—a soft blue satin dress by Jessica McClintock. She just so happened to find it at the same dress shop Gabby had bought her wedding dress only a few years earlier.

Before taking the gown home, Grace tried it on for a final check. She came out of the dressing room with a smile that stretched across her face. She looked absolutely stunning.

Grace stood on the raised platform where she could see herself in all the angled mirrors. The long gown had a modest halter top with a low back, fitted tightly through the waist and flaring to the floor. Silver heels peeked out from underneath the hem. Grace twirled and watched the fabric float around her.

Maureen took a deep breath, trying to find words to articulate how beautiful her daughter looked.

"You look breathtaking," she finally said.

"Thanks, Mom. Do you think Brandon will like it?" Grace replied as she held her hair up and then swooped it to one side, mentally deciding how she would wear it on prom night.

"More than your father will appreciate, I'm afraid," Maureen said as she winked at Grace. "Now go on, you better get changed. We still have so much to do before Friday night."

Grace came out of the dressing room a few minutes later in her jeans and sweater, ready for the next stop. With the dress hung safely in the backseat, they left for the florist to choose the boutonniere for Brandon's tux. He would be wearing a black suit with a white shirt and a blue tie and pocket accent for a pop of color to match Grace. *In my day, the whole tux would be baby blue. What were we thinking?* Maureen giggled at the thought.

At the florist, they choose a white rose with a blue edge for Brandon's tux. The place was jam-packed with girls choosing their dates' flowers and moms ordering corsages for their son's dates. Maureen glanced to her left and saw Brandon's mom, Stefanie, ordering flowers for Grace. *Uh oh*, Maureen thought as she intercepted Grace picking out her own flowers and shuffled her out the door to go home.

"But Mom! I just wanted..." Grace protested as she was being moved out the door.

"Nope, move along. Trust me; it is well taken care of, I'm sure. Moms have a special way of knowing these types of things," she said cryptically. Grace looked at her mom—who had a Cheshire Cat smile on her face—and gave in.

The next morning Maureen, Grace, and Rose all piled in the car and headed out at 9 a.m. for the salon with plans for a nice lunch afterwards. They had appointments to get their nails and toes done. It was their day to be pampered. Maureen looked forward to this day the most.

Even though they had appointments, they still got the obligatory "Pick a color. Ten minutes," as soon as they walked through the door. Maureen went there often and knew the girls. Their wait was only a few minutes before they were asked to sit in the massage chairs and soak their feet in the hot water bath.

Once Rose had gotten into her chair, Grace helped her get the massage set up to get the full experience.

"You are going to love this!" Grace said enthusiastically, setting up her own chair and leaning back to enjoy. Maureen loved watching them together.

Grace choose French tips for her fingers and a deep blue for the toes that would peek out from under her gown. Rose went for a short cut classic red on both, while Maureen did a mix of both—French tip on her fingers and red toes. Rose had never had a gel polish before, and it took her a while to get used to the drying machine used to set the gel. She had to have three fingers done twice.

The nail techs were exceptionally sweet and painted a single white flower on Rose's ring finger to remember Grant. Rose had shared stories about their lives the whole time they were there. Both Maureen and Grace listened intently and enjoyed the interpretations she added to what used to be relatively dull stories.

Maureen and Grace were both taken by surprise when they got back in the car and Rose admitted she had "spiced up her stories a bit." It still wasn't clear what part was spice and what part she felt was true, but neither of them asked. They all just laughed it off and went on their way to lunch.

They sat down for lunch at a new, hip farm-to-table place that Grace had been wanting to try—everything on the menu was organic and gluten-free. The atmosphere was warm with a natural palate, candles, and wine bottles for décor. They ordered goat cheese stuffed dates wrapped in bacon to start.

"They may be all natural, but these dates are sinfully good… and probably still filled with calories," Grace said as she popped another one into her mouth. The table had gone silent as they enjoyed the decadent appetizer. They decided to "splurge" a bit and ordered burgers with sweet potato fries and fish and chips to share.

Over lunch, they chatted about the rest of the week and decided that the next day, Wednesday, they would finalize accessories. Grace arrived home in the afternoon on Wednesday with her yearbook in hand. She was excited to look through it and show her family all the pictures she had made it into, but first focused on the finishing touches for prom.

Maureen and Grace sat down with Rose in the kitchen to talk about fashion and how best to accentuate the dress. Of course, Rose thought a hat would finish off the look perfectly.

"Oh honey, you would look like a movie star!" she said excitedly.

"Mom, Grace doesn't want to wear a hat to prom. She is having her hair done and wants to show it off," Maureen chimed in, coming to her rescue.

"I don't think I'll want to wear a hat, but there is something I would like to borrow," Grace offered, surprising both Maureen and Rose.

"And what would that be?" Maureen asked with one eyebrow raised, realizing that Grace had a plan.

"Wellll… when I was helping you unpack, I found a necklace that would be perfect!" she said, subconsciously holding her breath as she waited for the answer.

Rose knew just what she was talking about. It was the necklace Grant had given her for their 50th wedding anniversary. She remembered showing it to Grace when they set up her jewelry box. The necklace was suspended in a blue Tiffany box. It was simple and elegant, a single blue sapphire teardrop that hung from a silver chain.

"Grace, you're right. It will be perfect," Rose said, surprising even herself. Grace let out the breath she had been holding while Maureen stood dumbfounded. She knew what the necklace represented, and letting Grace wear it for even a night was a huge deal for her mother.

"You will have to be soooo careful Grace," Maureen started to warn her, but Grace already had her arms around Rose. She quickly noticed tears welling up in Rose's eyes, and she knew it made her happy.

Maureen was a bit teary too. When she went to bed that night, she remembered when her father had presented the necklace at a dinner party. Their song played in the background as he slipped the sapphire around her neck and kissed her. They really did look like Bogart and Bergman. She fell asleep with this image in her mind.

When Maureen got up Thursday morning, Grace was getting ready to join her girlfriends to get spray tans. Living in Seattle didn't exactly lend itself to the natural glow they all wanted. Maureen waved goodbye and sat for a quiet cup of coffee.

As was expected, Friday's arrival was packed with activity. After a busy day of hair and makeup, Grace arrived back at the house to get ready for the big night. Maureen and Rose were there to help. Grace slipped on her dress and shoes, and Rose had the honor of putting the necklace on her. She gently lifted it from the blue box and stood behind Grace and fastened it around her neck.

"It is so beautiful," Grace gasped as she turned to hug Rose once more.

"Your grandfather would be so happy to see it on you tonight sweetheart," she said, holding Grace's face in her hands but being careful not to smudge her makeup. "You look like a shining star."

Grace waited upstairs for Brandon to come in the door so she could have a dramatic entrance. The idea came from Rose, and it worked. Brandon stood at the bottom of the stairs, looking sharp in his black tux. He gasped when he saw Grace coming down the stairs, but quickly put himself in check when he glanced over at Steve.

Despite the usual tough guy act that dads love to put on, both Steve and Maureen really liked Brandon. He would be going off to law school at UCLA in a few weeks, and they wondered how the transition would go for Grace.

"Remember, bring her back as you received her," Steve said to Brandon, both joking and serious.

"Yes, Sir," Brandon replied.

They took photos at the bottom of the staircase and left to go meet up with their friends.

"She looks like a movie star," Rose said to no one in particular after they left.

⚬

Carla had spent five days in England teaching on dementia and touring senior living residences before Clif joined her for some long overdue vacation time. Carla had found out that in the U.K., it is estimated that the cost of living with dementia is 2.6 billion pounds. There were so many people affected, and Carla had a desire to help as many as she could, but for the next few days, she would need to rest.

She checked into the Covent Garden Hotel, which was famous for the garden markets, the Royal Opera House, and street performers—none of which she had seen in her whirlwind days of work. Carla looked forward to Clif arriving and exploring the city together.

He arrived while she was at breakfast. The buffet was filled with large bowls of berries and melons, breads and pastries that would add a few extra pounds just by looking at them, and granolas surrounded by bowls of clotted cream, yogurt, nuts, and honey. There were also a variety of breakfast meats and eggs for the American travelers, knowing their taste buds in the morning were quite different. Carla knew Clif was set to arrive at any minute, so she fixed two plates and found a quiet corner for them to sit.

As soon as she sat down to sip some of her water, she spotted Clif walking towards her. "Honey, it is so good to see you!" she said, standing up to greet Clif with a hug and a long kiss. "I grabbed some breakfast for you before you go up to rest for a bit. Please, sit down—you have to be exhausted."

"I am, but seeing you makes it worth every minute," Clif said quietly as she smiled at him, holding his hand across the table.

He told her about his flight and the characters he met on the plane, pausing every once in a while to take a bite of food. He had chatted with a local couple who had given him a list of things to do, a young man who was moving to England to go to college abroad, and an elderly couple in the next row who was making a bucket list dream come true.

After finishing breakfast together, Clif went to their room to sleep for a few hours while Carla walked around the Covent gardens and enjoyed the flowers in bloom. She sat on a bench, taking in an astonishing variety of roses and wildflowers. England's official flower was the rose, and the Queen Elizabeth climbing roses covered many fences and walls, sending off a perfume that filled the air. England's diverse wildflowers surrounded her; the foxglove, Jacob's ladder, poppy, daffodil, heather, and mistletoe were among the many in the gardens.

Carla read in her book about the gardens that the native bluebell was Britain's most popular wildflower. They swayed in the morning breeze, creating a magical feeling as she drank tea and continued to read. *Clif and I will have to go to the Royal Garden while we are here,* Carla thought as she read about the million bulbs planted each year to bring it to life. It would rival the tulip festival they went to every year near Seattle.

Later that afternoon, after Clif had time to get some rest, Carla went to the room and gently woke Clif from his nap. They relaxed in the room together for a while before going out for the day. Today would be a slow, relaxing day exploring the full garden where Carla had spent her morning. After they were done enjoying the flowers, they planned to go see the Royal Opera House (as close to an opera as Clif would get), do some shopping at the garden markets and enjoy the many street performers they would run across along the way. Being foodies at heart, exploring the local restaurants was at the top of their travel must-do list. The couple Clif had met on the plane had recommended a couple hole-in-the-wall places to try out while they were here.

They spent the next two days getting to be full-blown tourists. They went to see the crown jewels at the Tower of London and the changing of the guard at Buckingham Palace, and spent a good chunk of time letting it all sink in. They enjoyed the little things most people might overlook, such as the red phone booths on the streets and the classic double-decker buses.

On their last night before heading home, they bought tickets to see *School of Rock* at the Gillian Lynne Theater, one of Andrew Lloyd Webber's newest theaters. They had scored amazing seats—front row in the first balcony. They had both watched the movie with Jack Black several times over the years, but the play took it to a whole other level. England's theater scene easily rivaled New York's. They indulged in cocktails in the hotel lobby after the play, dancing to music to live music and enjoying each other.

⁂

The house was packed to the brim for Grace's graduation, with most of the family coming in to celebrate. Gabby and Nash had flown in from Alaska and were staying at the house. Grant and Tiffany flew in as well but were staying at a hotel in the heart of the wine tasting scene in Woodinville. Josh had a few days off work and was home more often than usual to spend time with his sister and nephew. Everyone being there meant more work for Maureen, mostly cooking, but she wouldn't have it any other way. The only sibling that couldn't make it was Matt, who had to stay on base. Maureen knew he would be there in a heartbeat if he could, and Grace knew he was there in spirit.

Graduation was being held at the University of Washington on Friday evening at 7 p.m. Grace had to be there early and left in the afternoon on the transportation the school had arranged, cap and gown in hand.

Nash entertained Rose in the front room while everyone was busy getting things ready for the evening. He was fascinated with her. He had learned to walk and run since she had last seen him, and she was just as fascinated with him. Nash ran up to Rose and jabbered away, animated as always. He was pointing to some object he was interested in and squealing when Rose talked back to him as if she understood every word. He danced for her when music came on and grabbed her hand for her to do the same. She obliged, and they laughed together.

When Nash fell, Rose sang him a song she used to sing to Maureen and Grant as children. "Boom, boom, ain't it great to be crazy. Boom, boom, ain't it great to be nuts like we are. Funny and silly all day long. Boom, boom, ain't it great to be crazy." She sang it loud and as animated as she could, and Nash ate it up.

"We should record that and put it in one of those build-a-bears for Nash to take home," Gabby suggested. "He would love it! I wonder if they have a moose or a fox instead of a bear. That would fit his room perfect."

Maureen smiled, remembering her mom singing to her as a child. "That's brilliant, Gabby. We will do that before you fly home."

While Nash napped, Maureen, Rose, and Gabby went to the florist to pick up the bouquet of flowers they had ordered and a Hawaiian lei to give Grace after the ceremony. Tonight, it would be only family gathered to celebrate. They had planned to have another gathering on Sunday afternoon where friends would be joining.

The ceremony was long, but when Grace's name was called out, they forgot all about it. The family stood and hooped and hollered loud enough for her to hear crystal clear in the huge room. She turned to the direction of the sound and raised both hands in victory. *The last of my babies has graduated*, Maureen thought, both proud and nostalgic. She hugged Steve, and they congratulated themselves on their accomplishment of making it through one more.

Sunday afternoon quickly rolled around, and the house was filled with those coming to congratulate and celebrate with Grace. Steve manned the BBQ and Gabby had made cupcakes and fresh blueberry ice cream. "Thank God for the gift of electric ice cream makers," Maureen said to Gabby as she placed a second batch in the freezer.

It was an exceptionally warm day for Seattle, and everyone was dressed casually except Rose—who had on a cotton spring dress and sun hat to match. She was hosting, after all, and thought she should dress the part. Besides, the sun was out and she had to protect her face, so the hat made perfect sense. Of course, Maureen knew she would have worn a hat no matter what the weather.

Grant was busy dishing out college advice to Grace as he sipped a beer on the patio, and Maureen immediately saw the "someone please help me" look come across her face. Maureen casually walked up to them, tapping Grace on the shoulder and excusing herself for the interruption. "Grace, honey, Ang and Jimmy have arrived. You should go greet them."

"Thank you," Grace whispered as she moved over towards the food to hang out with her friends. She didn't want to be rude to her uncle, but she wanted to have fun with her friends. There was plenty of time to be serious and talk about her future but now wasn't her ideal time. She had been accepted to the University of Washington and would start in the fall. For now, her major was liberal arts, but she wasn't married to it just yet.

Grant turned his attention to Maureen and Rose. "Maureen, how is Mom doing? Is she taking her medications? She keeps telling stories and making things up. I thought the medication would help her memory. When I try to correct her, she gets mad and indignant with me. I am trying to keep her grounded. You certainly aren't."

"You're right Grant. I am not. By correcting her, you are calling her a liar. Who likes that? I have learned that there are some things you just have to go along with. What harm is in her stories being embellished? Grant, did you know that our mother was on a college rowing team? A winning rowing team, at that?" Maureen challenged Grant.

"What are you talking about? Are you believing her stories?" Grant replied, shaking his head.

"She was, and I would have never known had I not let her talk and left my judgement behind me. She has pictures of her on the team in those old albums we took home, but I believed her even before I saw them. We have a lot to learn." Maureen didn't usually stand up to her brother, but at that particular moment, she felt empowered. She needed him to know that she knew what she was doing and that their mom was doing perfectly fine.

"I... I didn't know... I just thought..." Grant started.

"That's right; you didn't know," Maureen interrupted. "You should be quiet for a change and take a chance to learn something."

Even at the cost of confrontation, Maureen felt liberated. She knew Carla would be proud of her for understanding Rose.

✺

Carla had spent most of her summer and into the fall writing her new book *Surviving Dementia for Families*. Between writing and speaking, she had been too busy to meet up with Maureen. They had texted and e-mailed several times, and Carla laughed out loud when Maureen described her conversation with Grant at Grace's graduation over an e-mail. *Families that are out of town often have an opinion about the life someone else is living.* She was glad Maureen stood her ground and had remembered and used some of the techniques she had learned in their visits. According to Maureen, Grant had spent some time listening to her after that.

Carla was currently preparing for the keynote presentation she was scheduled to give at the annual Ted Talk conference in Seattle. As she worked on her speech, she thought a lot about Maureen and Rose, the members of the audience at the television studio, and those she met in England. She had so many thought-provoking conversations with families across the country she had met at speaking engagements, as well as students she met studying various forms of dementia in medical classes, psychology, and social work. These young adults would form the care of the elderly in the future. She wanted to share with them her vision and see what they did with it.

Carla had a quest to teach, and this speech—this one 18-minute speech—had to be packed with practical information and techniques that the audience could take with them. It had to be profound enough to not only make an impact in their lives but something they would want to share with their circles as well. It would be recorded and saved as a YouTube video, which made it even more daunting. Carla took a deep breath and reviewed what she had so far, then began typing again.

∾

It was now fall, and Maureen had been planning a celebration for her 35th wedding anniversary for months. They had given up their Italy vacation when her mom moved in, and she wanted to show Steve how much it had all meant to her. She knew how sad he was that they weren't getting on a plane that week for the trip they had planned for years; creating Rose's guest suite had cost them their entire nest egg for the trip. He had been a good sport, but she knew deep down that he was disappointed.

She had made reservations at Altura, a fine Italian restaurant in Seattle. All their food was farm-to-table, and the menu changed with the seasons and availability of product. She had also booked a room at the downtown Hyatt for the evening. A staycation may be all they could have, but they were going to do it up right. Steve deserved it. They both did.

Josh drove Maureen to the hotel at noon so she could check in and get ready for the night. He didn't want any details. He had agreed to stay home and visit with Rose, and that was all he needed to know. His girlfriend, Natalie, was cooking dinner with Rose, learning her famous pasta sauce recipe. It was Italian all around.

Maureen checked into her room and stood in awe of the view she had been given. Knowing the plan, Gabby had sent a bottle of Maureen's favorite red wine by Brian Carter ahead of time, and it was waiting for her in the room along with a single violet rose in a bud vase. That was the flower from their wedding, and Gabby wanted the special touch to be there. She texted Gabby a thank you note before unpacking her bag. She had her hair done earlier in the day, so she sat back on the chaise lounge and rested for a moment, enjoying the quiet. That was a rarity for her these days. Steve wouldn't be joining her for a few hours so she could take her time getting ready. She opened the bottle of wine to let it breathe so she could have a glass later when she was putting on her makeup. She knew Steve wouldn't mind. Her eyes became more intense with a glass of wine.

Steve got ready at home. He went and had a haircut as well, and even agreed to a shave. He had never had it done before, but Josh insisted and had paid for the treat as his anniversary present. Between the hot shaving cream, a straight blade, and a hot towel afterward, he joked with Josh that the experience made him feel like he was famous or something.

Gabby was in charge of pampering their mom, and he took on Dad. Josh even picked out everything he would wear to dinner. Steve didn't know where they were going yet, but Josh was in on the surprise. Dressed up in a black suit with a blue shirt and black tie with small blue and white stripes, Steve left the family to pick up his bride.

Maureen put the last touches of her makeup on and looked around the room. Candles were already set out, ready to light after dinner, and she had brought her Echo to play Italian music. She would leave it playing so it greeted them when they entered later. The bed was turned down, and rose petals were spread out over the sheets—Maureen had seen that in a movie and thought it would be fun. A bottle of basil whiskey and two small glasses sat on the table in case they wanted a nightcap. She doubted they would, but she wanted the option just in case. It was Steve's favorite brand. She took one last glance in the mirror, dabbed on some perfume and went to the lobby to meet Steve.

Steve was standing by the lobby doors when he saw the elevator doors open, and Maureen emerged. It was like waiting for her at the altar all over again. She looked beautiful. Maureen wore a dusty blue silk dress that hit about mid-thigh. It hugged all the right places, and his heart beat a little faster at the sight of her black heels and the dress flowing about her. It came up around her neck and showed off her elegant bare shoulders. The simple diamond necklace he had given her years before hung around her neck. He half thought about skipping dinner and going straight to the room but knew better than to request it. He would enjoy the night first.

They had an amazing dinner—each plate looked like a work of art. Their appetizer was a parmesan crisp balanced on a wood block with prosciutto, figs, and honey scattered across it, followed by Branzino with wild herbs cooked in butter, wine and garlic over wild rice. Broccolini laid perfectly on the side of the plate, framing the entire course. For dessert, they shared cheesecake. It was quite simple, with a drizzle of a bourbon caramel sauce spread perfectly underneath and fresh whipped cream on top. They spent hours at dinner, enjoying every minute of the food, atmosphere and each other. It was as if time stopped all around them, and reminded them of the simplicity of a beautiful marriage: they were in it together, through thick and thin.

They returned to the room, opening the door to the romantic sounds of Italian music playing and rose petals scattered. We'll keep the rest of the night a secret only they know...

Chapter Nine

*M*aureen sunk into her favorite chair in the living room. The air was chilly, and Steve had made a fire to cozy the room as they enjoyed a glass of wine and a quiet evening. The look on Maureen's face spoke to a melancholy, introspective mood as she sipped her wine.

"Are you ready for a slice of cake with those thoughts?" Steve prodded her with a smile.

"Oh yeah," she started, snapping out of her daze. "Sorry, I was just thinking about how much life has changed over the last year. Thank you for all your support honey. I know it hasn't always been easy, but knowing you are by my side has eased the tough times. There have been some great times too." Maureen smiled at Steve as he handed her a generous slice of vanilla cake with chocolate frosting she and Rose had made earlier that evening.

Balancing his cake and glass of wine, Steve settled into his chair. "It wasn't the year we had planned a year ago, but you're right, we are as strong as ever. Life sure has been an adventure."

"To whatever comes our way, together," they said in unison, clinking their glasses together for a toast. It had become their motto over the past year, and the thought of being together through whatever came their way kept them grounded.

Maureen's phone chimed as a text came in. She picked up her phone, read the text and shot off a response. "Work?" Steve asked. "Yes, a new patient was having a hard time understanding why she had to stay there this afternoon. They were letting me know she is calmed down and resting without the need for medication. We have certainly come a long way at work too," Maureen said as she looked at the emoji of a sleepy face that her team had sent back to her.

Maureen had changed floors at the hospital, and instead of working with the general population, she was now on a primarily geriatric floor. Maureen was able to practice the skills Carla had taught her, and she was teaching them to the other nurses and caregivers as well. The team on that floor had strengthened communication among themselves and were proud of the fact that they had reduced the use of medications with patients who were confused. It took a little more time and work, but, in the end, it was a win for everyone. Her supervisor had taken notice and had made Maureen a team lead for the nurses.

"What was her story?" Steve asked, curious about the patient. He knew there would be a story and that Maureen would have flushed it out to help her.

Maureen began, "She came up to be admitted from the emergency room after a bad fall. No broken bones, but she was dehydrated and had pneumonia. She was agitated in the ER, and they had given her the medication Haldol to calm her down. After the meds, she was more passive for sure, but still not calm. She kept worrying about her 'baby,' and everyone believed she was demented. An 80-something-year-old woman does not normally have a baby, so they didn't question it any further. Apparently, her family had been notified of her fall from the alert pendant she wore and were on their way to the hospital. However, they hadn't arrived yet when she got to my floor."

"Once we got her situated in a room, she was still restless. She was calling out for 'baby' and trying to get up. The caregiver came and let me know, so I followed her back to the room to see how I could help her. The patient had an order for additional medication, but I didn't want to give that to her yet." Steve drank his wine while he watched Maureen tell the story. He loved hearing the confidence and passion in her voice.

"She watched me as I entered the room. You could see she didn't trust anyone at this point. I calmly introduced myself and asked how I could help her. I shared that I understood she was worried about her 'baby,' and that the caregiver had brought me in to help. I don't think she trusted me yet, but she calmed down a bit when I sat at her bedside and waited for her to talk to me. She fell back into the same agitation as in the ER, raising her voice a bit as she urged that she had to go home to take care of her baby. He needed her. He would be scared. She then asked where her son was. It took all I had not to add to her story or ask about specific facts, but I knew I needed to let her guide the story. I remembered the techniques I had been using with Rose and prompted her to keep talking by asking her to tell me about the baby, matching her tone of voice to show I heard her concern. 'They locked him in the bathroom,' she started. Knowing I was listening, she then sighed deeply and told me about 'baby'—her 5-year-old Yorkie the ambulance drivers had put in the bathroom when they came and took her to the hospital. Baby never left her side, and she knew he must be confused and scared." Maureen had a big grin on her face by this time. "I let out my own breath at that revelation, not even realizing that I had been holding it. I assured her that her family was on their way and that we would make sure that her son checked on Baby as soon as they saw she was alright. She laid back in her bed, closed her eyes and finally rested.

"I could understand why the staff thought she was so confused. It took a while for her to get the whole story out to me, and I made sure I wasn't rushed. Her words were jumbled at times, but as she relaxed, she was much better. Her children got there a few minutes later and confirmed that she did have some short-term memory issues, but was still successful living on her own. Her son reassured her he would go care for Baby, and that she would be home in a few days to see him herself. She got a bit restless again in the afternoon as my shift was ending, still worried about Baby. The caregiver had a great idea: we should request that her son send us a video of Baby playing at his house with the grandchildren. He sent it over, and seeing Baby on the phone seemed to help. They showed it to her again this evening. It worked better than any medication. We all loved watching the video with her too." Maureen beamed with pride at the innovative thinking her team had demonstrated.

"Sounds like you made a big difference in that person's life. I am so proud of the way you have taken everything you have learned about dementia and applied it to your work life," Steve spoke with admiration for his wife.

"I have an opportunity coming up to teach a class for the ER team as well. When my supervisor heard about how we handled this situation, he asked me to speak on dementia at the next staff meeting with the ER team. I am excited to share what I know. I know this is just the beginning, but I hope this class helps change the way seniors are looked at when they come into the ER, at the very least. They have to move fast in the ER, I get that, but in some ways, that is taking more time." Maureen thought for a moment before finishing. "I hope we can hold off on scheduling the class until after I hear Carla give a TED Talk at the end of the month. That will give me more to share."

"Is Grant still coming to hear Carla as well?" Steve inquired.

"Yes, he is. I am going to keep it a surprise for Mom though, in case his plans change," Maureen gave Steve a wink and a smile.

Steve refilled their wine glasses and took away the plates that had once held the cake. As he entered the kitchen, he asked, "Are Brandon and Natalie still joining us for dinner tomorrow night?"

"Yes, I thought it would be nice to have him over before he leaves for school. Grace is going to be heartbroken when he goes. Since Brandon was coming over, I told Josh to ask Natalie as well. Two children and their dates, you, me and Mom," Maureen explained. "I thought we could have Mom's fried chicken, potatoes and a green salad. The chicken is already marinating in buttermilk."

"Sounds great to me. I am making the potatoes, right?" Steve asked to clarify. "Remember the last time Rose made them? She added hot water from the pot to mash them, and they tasted like water," Steve made an overexaggerated face to make his point. "I know she was trying to keep them hot, but they weren't really edible." Maureen laughed remembering that first bite of potatoes. It was comical to look around at everyone's faces trying to act like they were delicious so as not to hurt Rose's feelings. "Yes, you are in charge of the mashed potatoes. We will heat up the milk a bit so mom doesn't worry about them being cold. Lots of butter too. I know I am a nurse and should eat healthily, but what are mashed potatoes without pools of real butter on top right before serving? Yummmmm, so good," Maureen said, licking her lips at the thought.

"There won't be any cake left after the kids get home and see it," Steve said with a twinkle in his eye. His smile told Maureen exactly what he was asking for. "Peach pie for dessert?" she asked, knowing full well what he wanted was apple. Steve made a face and Maureen laughed. "OK, apple it is."

"For that, you get a dance."

Jon Pardi's *Head over Boots* had come on the radio. Steve held out his hand, and Maureen took it with pleasure. A little country two-step in the kitchen reminded Maureen of her parents dancing in the kitchen in the evenings when she was young. Steve spun Maureen around the room over and over and gave her a dramatic dip at the end. They laughed and danced to another song. It was a simple thing, but they both knew nights like this were special; something almost out of a Hallmark movie. *I guess my mom and I are a lot alike,* Maureen thought as she spun around the kitchen floor to music on Amazon and a fire roaring in the fireplace.

The peace and quiet gave way to the reality of young adults as Grace, Brandon and their friends, Jimmy and Angi, came through the door. "Mind if we watch a movie?" Grace asked. "Go ahead, enjoy. There's cake on the counter," Maureen replied. She was about to add "Save a slice for Josh" when he and Natalie came through the door. "I guess we are the place to be," Maureen said to Steve as the kids got comfortable on the couches and floor.

⌁

The next morning, the house was quiet as Maureen came downstairs. The kids had done a fairly good job cleaning up after themselves, and as Steve had predicted, the cake was gone.

Steve had a morning job and came down to have a cup of coffee with Maureen before they both had to leave. Maureen had a staff meeting with her team and had a few things to check on before getting home.

The staff meeting was held in a small conference room on the geriatric floor where Maureen worked. The nurses and caregivers came together once a month to review successes and opportunities and have an in-service on any number of topics. Maureen had been teaching the staff members the same communication skills and techniques that she had learned from Carla, and she was proud to see them implemented on the floor. She wrote out cards to encourage and thank each one for taking the lessons seriously. Each time she saw someone do something that illustrated their new-found knowledge, she took note and wrote out a recognition card. Writing the cards were the highlight of her day. She had taken everything Carla had taught her and passed on that knowledge to her staff. She was really proud of each and every one of them, and couldn't wait to tell Carla about all that they were accomplishing. She also knew she would have so much more to share with them after hearing Carla speak in a few weeks.

The room quickly filled up with nurses and caregivers, the sound of their chatter echoing through the halls. They knew Maureen always started on time, and she always had treats ready to enjoy. Today was no exception. The table they sat around had bowls of nuts, chips, hummus, cheese curds, small pastries and chocolate waiting to be devoured. The staff filled their plates and sat back quietly in their seats as Maureen got started.

"Good morning! In the last month, I have had so many opportunities to see you using the techniques I've taught. I decided to write cards for each of you to commend the effort you have put into learning more about your patients and using amazing listening skills. I wrote so many that my hands started to hurt! Please pass them around the room." Maureen held up a stack of thank you cards and let them drop on the table. There was one for everyone in the room, and some had multiple cards as Maureen had seen them demonstrate these skills multiple times. As they passed the cards around, she made sure to verbally acknowledge each one. "I'd like to recognize Pam for taking a deep breath and getting focused before entering each room to be able to be fully with each patient, Mitch for calming a patient down by talking about the blueberry fields the patient had grown up in before starting care, and Sean for finding the right channel on the TV so his patient felt at home and could sleep to the sound of familiar voices."

Maureen went on with story after story. "Lastly, I'd like to recognize Phallon, who thought out of the box to ask a patient's son to video her dog, Baby, playing with the grandchildren and send it to us so we could play it at any time she was missing her 'baby.'" The room broke out in applause with every story. "You are all learning about your patients and using that information to help them get well faster. Each of you are what makes this hospital, this floor, and this team great. You are who the families see as the hospital. The fancy equipment and rooms are anywhere. It is *you* who make a difference."

As the meeting was ending, Maureen's supervisor, Derek, stopped in to say hello to the team. "Great job this past month team. Your patient reviews have been amazing. I know that Maureen writes a lot of thank you cards each month to you for the special care you give, and it is about time she gets one back." Derek handed Maureen a card signed by all her staff along with a small bouquet of flowers.

"Thank you, each of you. I am touched," Maureen said, wiping a tear from her eyes. "OK, come on now, we have patients to see," she said quickly to stop herself from crying more. "I will see you all in a couple days. Call if you need anything." Maureen left the hospital and headed home, smiling all the way.

Chapter Ten

*F*rom backstage, Carla peeked out at the audience for the TED Talk. The auditorium was packed with thousands of professionals from all around the country, Seattle locals from all walks of life, and aspiring speakers waiting for the day that they would be on the stage. Currently, a naturopath was talking about the use and abuse of vitamins and supplements. The audience appeared to be hanging on to every word she spoke.

Even though Carla had spoken in front of large crowds before and had been on TV and radio, she found herself to be a bit more nervous than she had felt in the past. She found a small, quiet space backstage to get centered. Carla took several deep breaths, letting each out slowly. As she did so, her nerves calmed, and she was ready to focus on educating and captivating the audience before her. She hoped to bring something that would not only go on to change the lives of the people in the room, but all who would watch the replay on the TED Talk network in the future.

Carla had dressed in her favorite deep violet suit. The slightly flared skirt came to mid-calf and had a high waist that made her midsection look smaller than it was. Like any woman, that always made Carla happy. The jacket met the skirt at the waistband. Under her jacket, she wore a silk blouse in a simple cream color. She wore black velvet heels that looked elegant, and only Carla knew they were also exceptionally comfortable. She smoothed her hair and touched up her makeup one last time before stepping up to be called next on stage.

"Please welcome to the stage, Carla Veloza!" the announcer's introduction boomed, bringing Carla to life. She walked on the stage, acknowledged the audience, and thanked the announcer before turning her full attention to her audience with a smile. She took a deep breath and dove in.

"When I was a child, receiving a cancer diagnosis was the greatest fear anyone could have. Many of my own family members received that diagnosis. All but one of them died." She let the last word hang in the air.

"Today there is a diagnosis that creates even greater fear. That is the diagnosis of Alzheimer's."

Carla gracefully glided across the stage, speeding up a bit. "In the United States today, there are 5.7 million people diagnosed with Alzheimer's. Two-thirds of those are women, and 200,000 are under the age of 65. It is the sixth leading cause of death in the United States. From 2000 to 2015, the death rate from Alzheimer's rose 123%."

Carla took a slow, deliberate breath and stood still on the stage. "It is incurable and unrelenting, leaving families without the key to communicate. I am here today to give you that key."

As Carla continued to speak, she captivated her audience with her passion. "Some time ago I sat in an apartment with an elderly widow. Her husband had passed a year earlier. She needed care assistance, and I agreed to meet with her son to talk to her. The woman sat in a small winged-back chair in a one-bedroom apartment within an assisted living community. Her white hair was combed neatly into place, and a small barrette held bangs away from her eyes. She looked quite frail. We chatted for a time about her life in the community and her favorite activities. She liked music and a glass of wine at happy hour. I wanted her to be comfortable before talking about more personal things. As we talked, the woman looked about the room as if she were looking for something, for someone.

"'Where is my husband?' the woman asked. Before I could respond, her son interrupted with deep anguish in his voice. 'Mom, Dad is dead. Don't you remember? He died a year ago.' The woman crumpled into her lap and sobbed her eyes out. For her, it was like hearing it for the first time. Her heart broke, and she mourned deeply for him. Seeing her in pain broke the son's heart as well."

Carla moved back from storyteller to educator as she stood still once more. "We have been taught since we were young to never lie to your parents. It was the biggest offense you could make, and their trust in you could be lost. Yet, here, in this instance, telling the truth causes pain for everyone involved.

"This tension is called reality orientation. Reality orientation is, simply put, 'the facts.' For example, 'Today is Monday,' or 'The city is Manhattan.' In the story above, it starts with 'Your husband is…'" Carla shook her head. "When I started in this field nearly 30 years ago, we planned to start each day through reality orientation with our patients. We would make sure to ask them what day of the week, month, year, or season it was. If they couldn't remember, we would tell them again and again. As if knowing this all held some importance we never understood. According to the State, it was essential in every care plan. Thank goodness times have changed. Groundbreaking understanding in the last few decades has taught us that none of those details are important when dementia is present. Their truth and ours are just different, and that's OK.

"When we challenge a person's truth, we are essentially calling them a liar. We are telling them they don't know the information they feel passionate about. I don't know about you, but I'm guessing you don't like being called a liar or uninformed any more than I do." The audience laughed. "That's what I thought. Neither do they.

"Let me share another technique that is still taught to caregivers today, called 'The Therapeutic Lie.' In this scenario, the son may have said, 'Mom, Dad is at work. He will be here later.' He is trying to pacify her for the time being, hoping she will forget the question he doesn't want to have to answer. What harm is there in that? This 'therapeutic lie' may calm her down for the time being, and he can avoid upsetting her." Carla paused, looking around the room to see and acknowledge some of the audience members nodding their heads in agreement.

"Can you tell when someone is lying to you? Do you like it? Do you trust those who lie to you?" The question silenced the audience, and they sat still, each knowing their answer deep down. "Those with dementia can deeply feel your emotion. They may not know you're lying, or what the lie is directly related to, but they know something isn't right. Furthermore, the question still lives on in their mind. It may disappear for a moment, but it will most likely be back.

"By now I'm sure you might be asking, 'If I can't do all those things, then what CAN I do? How do I answer the question that pains us all?' Well, I have a solution for you." Carla watched as the audience sat forward, waiting to hear her answer.

"When I get asked the question, 'Where is my husband?' I answer in one of two ways. The first is to ask them about him: 'Tell me about your husband.'

"I have found that when someone asks this question, they either have a memory floating up or are feeling a need for the person at that moment. In the story I told earlier, the woman was under stress—she was talking to a stranger who was asking questions, and she didn't know how to answer them, so she looked for her husband for help. By asking the simple question, 'Tell me about your husband,'" Carla reiterated, "the woman would be able to share a thought or memory of him. The conversation would shift to her memories, and she could share whatever came up—true or not—allowing the thought to pass.

"This detour may take some time but will give you so much more information than any other question you could ask. It would let me know her belief about her husband, which is something important to her, and where she was living in her memories. There is nothing more important than those pieces of their life. Keep asking the same question with a slight variation as you move through the conversation—'Tell me about your house, home, children, etc.'—whatever IT is. I have heard the best stories by asking these sorts of questions. I don't know what percentage of the stories were accurate, but I also didn't care. They were having a conversation with me, and they felt in control and important. It was a gift to them, and a blessing to me."

Carla changed gears a bit, lowering her voice. "There are times when they are sharing a memory and talking for a bit, and will suddenly stop mid-sentence. They look at you and say something like, 'You know my husband died? I miss him.' Reality drifted up through the jumble of tangled thoughts that the disease has plagued them with. At this point, you should acknowledge their loss and let them talk about it.

"As caregivers, and as people, we have a desire to help others feel better. We are not comfortable with grief, yet it needs to be acknowledged. It is an emotion we have all experienced and can relate to." Carla paused, giving a chance for the weight of her words to sink in. "Who listened to you when you needed to talk? Be that person for them," she said, glancing around the room. "By listening, we allow for a resolution to begin and peace to come in. They don't always remember things like this, but it is important to be prepared if it does."

Carla moved across the stage again as she shifted gears once more. "Now for the second way to answer the question." She could see they were ready to hear more. "The second question I might ask is, 'It is 10 a.m. on a Thursday. Where would your husband be on a Thursday at 10 a.m.?' I often get an answer such as, 'He'd be at work, of course.' You might get the *How stupid are you, lady?* look." Carla gave the audience the same animated look she had received in the past, and they laughed. "I follow that with, 'Tell me about his work.' See, I'm using that *tell me* question again. Then you listen and learn again. It is a circle of conversation."

In closing her talk, Carla tied it up nicely for them. "Communicating isn't rocket science. It is simple after you throw out a few rules. Slow down. Taking an extra five minutes to listen to a story is priceless. I ask you to let go of reality. Let your mind be open to accepting *their* beliefs. Let *them* lead you in a conversation, even if it doesn't make perfect sense or couldn't possibly be true. Once you let go, you let them in. It will change their lives."

Carla gave a slight bow and said, "Thank you." The audience clapped, many of them standing. Carla looked across the audience, smiled warmly, nodded a thank you and left the stage.

Once backstage, Carla walked past the set-up area and back through the halls to the prep room where she collapsed in a chair. She had mustered up every ounce of passion and energy she had and left it out on that stage. She was pleased. She had about 30 minutes to relax before she had to make her way into another room with the vendors to sell her new book and greet members from the audience. Her children, Christian and Twila, had been manning her table for a couple hours already, but she knew that the next break would be when people would be more interested in meeting her. She wanted to be able to greet them. Dementia was personal to her. She felt the need to give that personal touch back to her audience and readers.

The large vendor auditorium held more than 50 booths, all centered around health. Carla arrived right before the next break started. She took a loop around the room to take it all in and stopped to talk with a few of the other speakers she had heard earlier in the day. The vendors represented ranged from doctors advertising their practices to people selling essential oils, to information on the latest diet, to medical equipment. There was new technology everywhere: booths that had wheelchairs that climbed stairs and necklaces that had GPS to track where a person was and would call for help in case of a fall. There was even full smart house technology for the elderly that "learned" a person's patterns and called if there was unusual behavior. There were naturopaths, massage therapists, and natural healers of all types. People were walking about the building visiting different tables, and a soft murmur ran through the room. The crowd would be light until the break started in a few minutes. Carla got comfortable in a chair at her table with a bottle of water to keep her hydrated. Christian and Twila sat with her, enjoying a few moments before the next wave of people came in. She loved having her children at her side at such events. They chatted for a minute or two before they looked up just in time to see the crowd pouring into the room like ants at a picnic. *Here we go.* The murmur started to become a roar.

For the next 90 minutes, Carla signed copies of her book and gave bits and pieces of insight to those who came armed with a question. It was a whirlwind of activity; much more than she had anticipated. She wasn't going to bring many books with her, but Twila had argued, "Mom are you kidding me? We are taking as many as I can get in the car." Twila was managing the table, so Carla didn't argue with her after she insisted.

After all the commotion settled, they went to pack the books back into the car. To Carla's surprise, all that was left was able to fit into one box. "Thank you for not listening to me," Carla said as they cleaned up. "Mom, we do listen to you. That's why I knew. They were listening too," Twila cocked her head toward the crowd that was slowly filtering out to their cars. Carla looked at her children and beamed with appreciation and affection.

"Thank you, my children. Love you."

"We know" they both said, and she hugged them.

⬧

Maureen had bought the ticket to the TED Talk event as soon as she had heard Carla would be speaking. She even convinced Grant to go with her. It was a big step for him, and she knew that. She also knew he needed it—more than he would ever admit. To her surprise, he wanted to sit through all the talks. For her, the cost of the ticket—no cheap seats here—was worth it even if she only heard Carla speak. To Grant, the price meant you have to take it *all* in.

Grant was deep in his analytical mind as he listened to the speakers. He commented on whether he thought their ideas were worthwhile or not, and engaged Maureen in banter about several nursing topics. However, it all changed when Carla hit the stage. The main event had begun.

Grant quickly became quiet when Carla walked onstage. He even appeared to soften a bit. Maureen wasn't sure why, but she took it as a good sign. He listened intently and nodded his head as Carla spoke. When Carla described the elderly woman in the apartment asking about her husband, Grant took Maureen's hand and squeezed it, and held on. Maureen was both shocked and pleased at the same time. In those last 18 minutes, he never let go of her hand. They nodded in agreement together, laughed, and tears filled their eyes thinking about what was to come in their future. It was the closest Maureen could ever remember them being. At the end, as Carla walked off, he squeezed her hand again, looked at her, and simply said, "Thank you."

When the next speaker came on, Grant returned to his intellectual, analytical self again. However, Maureen saw him glance at her a couple times from the corner of her eye, and she knew he was still processing his feelings.

During one of the breaks, Maureen finally got to ask Grant about Carla's talk. "Grant, thank you for coming. I wondered what made you say yes." Grant looked at the ground for a moment and then admitted to her that he had been listening to her talk to their mom each time he called after the graduation party where she "set him straight."

"I went out and bought one of Carla's books. It made sense to me. Practical. I wanted to actually... *hear her live*. It was definitely worth it."

⊸

It had been over a year since Carla had seen Maureen *and* Rose. She had kept in contact with Maureen over time, and had briefly spoken for a moment at the TED Talk event. Carla was surprised to see Grant there but was flattered that he had come. He had bought her new book, and she signed it like he was an old friend. She wrote:

> *Grant,*
> *Thank you for embracing Rose and her life as she shares it.*
> *Carla.*

Through texts, e-mails and a few phone calls from Maureen, Carla knew about Grace's prom and graduation, Maureen standing up to Grant at the graduation party, and even heard about the Italian anniversary date. Carla had kept Maureen up to date about England, and had been in touch as she wrote the book that was released at the TED Talk.

Sitting in the same coffee shop where she and Maureen had met after the television show, Carla watched with anticipation for the two to arrive. Three soft chairs were set close by the fireplace around a wood table. Carla had ordered a mocha and was taking her first sip when she saw them arrive. She smiled brightly, setting the drink down on the table.

She saw Maureen first. She looked good, as if she had settled into a rhythm in life. She appeared to stand taller yet looked relaxed as she did. Her jeans were tucked into riding boots with a soft blue mid-thigh length sweater. Rose was, well, Rose. She had on a blue dress that was cinched at the waist with a wide blue belt. A matching hat perched on her head, smaller this time but still holding the classic 1940's look. Her hair formed soft waves around it. Rose still wore heels, although Carla noticed that they were a little shorter this time.

They stepped into the café and went right to Carla. "Of all the gin joints in all the towns in all the world, she walks into mine," Rose quipped from Casablanca as soon as she saw Carla and winked. Rose gave her a big hug like a long lost relative, and Maureen joined in before going over to order coffee and pastries.

Rose was as animated as ever as she shared her stories with Carla. They all drank coffee and nibbled on quiche and pastries as conversation moved along. Rose told her how stunning Grace was at prom, "The sapphire necklace brought it all together. Movie star quality," she said proudly. She told stories of cooking pasta with Josh and playing with Nash during the holidays when Gabby and Matt had come down for a few days. She even sang Carla the "Boom Boom song" she now sang to Nash every time they called. Carla noted that a few more words were hard for Rose to find as she talked, and the stories had more embellishment when she couldn't remember the story exactly as it happened. There was a small decline in communication in those moments, but nothing that completely stopped the conversation. If you were willing to listen, she was willing to talk.

Maureen was able to get a few words in when Rose took an infrequent breath between stories. She told Carla that she had a new focus at work, and would be leading a floor that was primarily for the elderly. Maureen was asked to consult with those with dementia on a regular basis. Her supervisor had watched her using the techniques that she had learned from Carla over the past year and was impressed with how patients had responded to her. "I have so much empathy for families with parents who have dementia. I share my story and encourage them to be open. The gift shop at the hospital now stocks your books, by the way. I send a lot of people there to buy them," Maureen shared, spilling over with her excitement about this new adventure.

"Do I owe you royalties?" Carla teased.

"Nope. Just more books and coffee, with pastries of course," Maureen replied, and they shared a good laugh before Rose took off on another story.

While Rose left them alone for a bit to go to the restroom, Maureen took the time to find out how Rose was doing at the house. In addition to having trouble with communication, Rose was having more difficulty with the remote—any technology, really—although she managed to play her brain games on the iPad still. At least until she pushed the wrong button and it disappeared until someone came home and got the game back up. She was only allowed to walk to the store with someone else, and only on sunny days, which were a rare occasion in Seattle. Things always seemed to go "missing," but eventually turned up in the most interesting places. Many things found their way into the freezer—everything from measuring cups to wallets. It became the first place they looked whenever anything was missing. They had some tough days, but overall, they were making it through.

What she had learned was working well for her right now, but Maureen knew that wouldn't always be the case.

"What's next, Carla? What do I have to prepare for as we move forward?" Maureen asked quietly.

"Take things one day at a time. Everyone moves from one stage of dementia to another at different paces and exhibit different behaviors along the way. There will be days when you wonder if the confusion was just a bad dream and other days that try your patience. It is a bit like a rollercoaster. Learn to cherish the good days. It will help you through those that are more difficult. I hope you know you can reach out to me at any time to get direction," Carla reassured her.

Rose was approaching the table, and Carla reached out and squeezed Maureen's hand much as Grant had done during the talk. "You don't have to do it alone," she said tenderly. Maureen could see through the compassion on her face that those words were more than true on Carla's end, and she could also see it playing out in her family as well. After the Ted Talk, Grant was more open to conversations, and the entire family was willing to offer support in any way they could.

Steve was always there for her, and he helped her remember his favorite lesson from the Sandwich Generation: to remember to take care of yourself as the caretaker. He planned getaways for them on a regular basis, although Maureen knew that he was trying to capture some of the time they were missing. She smiled at the thought. Steve had given up so much since her mother had moved in: their trip to Italy, being an empty nester after Grace went off to college, and being able to pack up and go away on a whim. Everything took planning nowadays. Maureen loved Steve even more for all he did for her.

Maureen turned her attention back to the conversation, and Rose was telling yet another story—this time about Nash. Nash had been drawn to Rose, and she was equally drawn to him. He listened to all her stories, and she listened intently to his, even if his idea of "talking" was mostly gibberish. They both were lively and animated and loved the attention.

A few hours flew by as they caught up, listening and laughing and learning from one another. The time to say goodbye came far too soon for their liking, but they each had to go their separate ways. As they hugged and made their way to the door, they promised to set another coffee date in the next month or so.

Maureen had started to walk toward the door with Rose trailing behind when Rose suddenly stopped and turned to look at Carla. In a classic Ingrid Bergman tone, Rose said, "I think this is the beginning of a beautiful friendship. Here's looking at you kid." Then she turned and left the shop, leaving Carla standing in her tracks smiling.

Definitions, Techniques, and Styles Used Throughout the Story

But first, one last thought for you.

Years ago, I heard an analogy from an anonymous author about how dementia feels as it progresses. The story is about a train ride. I have shared it here exactly as I have told it for the last ten years—my personal adaption of the original.

An elderly woman stood on the train platform clutching her purse as she waited for the train to arrive. She loved trains. Throughout her life, she rode the train to visit family and friends, and today she was going to see her children and grandchildren. She stared down the track in anticipation.

She soon saw the train in the distance and felt the ground rumble as it moved down the track to the platform. She heard the whistle blow as it pulled up in front of her.

"All aboard!" the conductor yelled out to welcome the passengers, and she eagerly boarded. She found a seat by a window and sat down. She looked around the train car, watching the families laughing as they got comfortable. Their smiles made her feel warm and happy.

Suddenly, she felt herself get pushed into the seat as the train sped up quickly, leaving the station. She looked out the window and watched the familiar farms and towns she knew pass by her. She enjoyed the scenery as it slipped by, with big oak trees lining the way and lots of cows. The low rumble of the train and its movement soon lulled her to sleep.

When she awoke, she looked about the car and saw the passengers smiling, enjoying the ride and pointing out the windows at the scenery. She looked over at her own window but was surprised at what she saw outside. Nothing looked familiar to her anymore, and she grew concerned. There were no farms or towns, and the trees didn't look right to her. *I must be on the wrong train. This isn't right. I have to get off,* she thought.

Her heart started to beat faster as she stood and looked about the train once again. She spotted an exit door and began to move toward it. A car attendant saw her move toward the exit and stopped her.

"Ma'am, can I help you?"

"I have to get off the train. I am going the wrong way. I have to leave."

Her heart was beating faster still, and she wanted to cry. The attendant smiled at her and took the ticket she had been clenching in her hand.

"Ma'am, you are on the right train. Now let me help you back to your seat. Everything is fine. I will tell you when we get to your stop."

She wasn't sure, but he seemed so nice and reassuring. His smile was warm and calming. He spoke to her in a kind voice, and although she didn't understand everything he was saying, she trusted him and sat back down. He smiled at her again and then moved down the aisle.

She sat back in her seat and looked again around the room. The people on the car seemed fine, but she thought it was odd that they didn't speak much English. *Weren't they speaking English before?* She didn't look out the window again but watched the passengers for a bit more before the train again lulled her to sleep.

This time when she woke up, she felt anxious. Something didn't feel right. She looked out the window again and this time what she saw horrified her. The familiar scenery was replaced with trees that were ugly and misshapen. She gasped and stood up to run.

Strong arms grabbed her as she ran to the door. She fought them, but couldn't get away. "Please let me go. I must get off the train. Please let me go!" she wailed. She feared she would never get to her children. They needed her, and she was being taken away from them.

The attendant and another man took her back to her seat. "Calm down and sit. You are fine. We will tell you when you can get off. This guard will be right here to make sure you stay put until we get to your stop," he said firmly. His smile had been replaced with frustration and annoyance. She had lost all control. *He will tell me... He doesn't know me. How can he tell me?* Tears now streamed down her face.

A few hours later she cried and called out for help, but no one came. The people around her looked at her sympathetically but stayed away. She tried once more to get up, but the man held up his hand and wouldn't let her go.

Where are they taking me? Will my children ever be able to find me? What will happen when we stop? Oh, how I want my husband. Where is he? Thoughts raced and rambled through her mind; some staying for a bit and others leaving as fast as they came.

She sat back in her seat and drew quiet. She waited, rocking herself like her mother had when she was scared. She looked out the window once more, but this time saw nothing.

This is what it may feel like as someone moves through the various stages of Alzheimer's and their understanding of the world around them fades away. At first, everything feels and looks comforting and reassuring, but as time goes by and the disease progresses what was once familiar becomes confusing. The reality they are living in and the reality in their minds are in conflict. Being unable to reconcile the conflict creates fear. These are the times when you hear "I want to go home," or "Where is my husband?" as they search for comfort. When confronted with continued reality, such as "You live here now," or "Your husband died," they withdraw from those around them. However, if you join them in their reality, you bring them peace. *"Tell me about your home, your husband."* Listen, really listen, and allow them to find comfort in their stories.

Signs of Dementia

Chapter One through Four

In the first four chapters of this book, I laid out a sample of possible signs of dementia that a family may want to give more attention to. We all forget names, misplace our keys or forget to turn off the oven. However, when these signs are seen together consistently, something far more serious may be occurring. The following is in no way a complete list, and more can be found on the Mayo clinic website at: mayoclinic.org.

In this story, the signs shown were:

1. Pearls being found in the silverware drawer when Rose had always kept them in a special place in her jewelry box

2. Notes placed all around the house to remind Rose of everything

3. Maureen's gut feeling that something was not right

4. Rose repeating lines from Casablanca throughout the book when it had only been between her and her husband in the past

5. Burning food when normally an excellent cook

6. Calling family several times a day and night

7. "Missing" items that are blamed on someone for taking them or hiding them from her

8. Hiding belongings and then not remembering where they are

9. Repeated calls to 911 that are for trivial things or unfounded fears

10. Not understanding the smoke detector alarm

11. Unable to use the remote or iPad, even when made simpler or shown repeatedly

12. Getting lost on walks and not admitting it; making up excuses

13. Establishing a routine and getting confused when it is interrupted

14. Overflowing the sink

15. Inability to remember how to load the dishwasher

16. Forgetting her purse and believing it was because the housekeeper moved it on her

17. Not having money with her to buy groceries

18. Bills that were previously paid in a timely manner are late or not paid at all

19. Giving away money to charities over the phone or in the mail

20. Telling stories that Maureen knew had never happened, but Rose was sure they did (or embellished a true story)

Here is a list taken from the Mayo Clinic website: https://www.mayoclinic.org/

Cognitive Changes

1. Memory loss, which is usually noticed by a spouse or someone else

2. Difficulty communicating or finding words

3. Difficulty reasoning or problem-solving

4. Difficulty handling complex tasks

5. Difficulty with planning and organizing

6. Difficulty with coordination and motor functions

7. Confusion and disorientation

Psychological Changes

1. Personality changes

2. Depression

3. Anxiety

4. Inappropriate behavior

5. Paranoia

6. Agitation

7. Hallucinations

Chapter Five

Additional signs of dementia from the story:

1. Worried that her husband wouldn't approve of the house sale as if he were still alive

2. Getting lost in the airport and needing an escort to get back

3. Rose's inability to get straight to where she was going in the airport, bouncing from one area to another to and from the restroom

4. Rose's free flow of stories with Carla on the plane and to anyone who would listen

In this story, we see that Rose's husband may have been hiding her forgetfulness from the children and taking on more to help her. There was also a possibility that they had been married for so long, that together they made a whole and any falters were brushed away as nothing.

Centering or Cleansing Breath

This tool is aimed at caregivers and is teaching the art of getting focused. This is often used in meditation to calm the voices of the world and get focused on you alone. Here we use it to quiet the world around us so we can give our undivided attention to the person we are speaking to. In Chapter 5, Carla takes a deep cleansing breath before starting the dementia conversation with Maureen on the plane. The technique of centering can be used at any time there is an emotional conversation, or you need to give someone your full attention.

In the centering I teach for beginners, I have you start by closing your eyes. Take a few deep, slow breaths, concentrating on each breath coming in and leaving your body. After a couple of these breaths, imagine a mist forming around you that you breathe in and watch in your mind as it blows out of your lungs. You can then change the mist to a color that is calming to you (for me I use lavender), then breathe it in again and blow it out a couple times. When your mind is quiet, slowly open your eyes.

After this exercise, you will feel peaceful and calm. After much practice, a single focused breath can bring you this achievement.

Hoarding

Holding onto items—lots of them— is commonly seen in all stages of dementia. This could include expired medications or magazines and newspapers that stack in corners and garages—things that never get looked at, but they can't seem to find peace in letting them go. It may be someone who has always collected things but recently got out of control, or it may be related to a death that is unresolved, so they symbolically "hold on" to items they still have.

In its worst state, hoarding can limit a person's ability to maneuver in a home with stacks blocking pathways creating possible fire hazards. Medication is common for a hoarder as it is costly and they "may need it again later."

For Rose, it was medication and magazines.

Panic

In the early stages of dementia, the person knows they are losing their memory and are getting confused by things that had previously been easy for them. We see this depicted in the fictional book "The Notebook" by Nicolas Sparks as well as the non-fiction "Still Alice" by Lisa Genova.

This is the same feeling you may get when you leave your home and can't remember if you turned off the oven. A panic sets in that takes over everything until you can figure out the answer. In these cases, there is an answer to find: you can go home or call a family member who can check for you, thus allowing yourself to let your fear go. With dementia, there isn't anything concrete to check to clear the feeling. They just know something is not right, and the feeling stays with them.

Assuming Best Intentions

It is important to remember that the person is doing the best they can with what they have available to them. I can assure you; they do NOT do things on purpose to bother or annoy you. Expect that each day will be different, and you will never be disappointed.

We all have good and bad days; days when things come easy and days when we get baffled by the simplest tasks. With dementia, these become amplified. The good days are great but the bad days are filled with emotion and frustration. For families, the good days give us hope, and we can fall back into believing that everything is fine, even when we know it is not. Then a bad day happens, and we grieve for our loss all over again.

Believe that who is in front of us today is doing their best that day and leave expectations for tomorrow behind us. Stay present, and it will be a blessing to you.

Slow Down

In this world today, we move at a fast pace and anticipate things even faster. A microwave—which years ago made our lives faster and easier saving us hours in the kitchen—seems to take too long for us. We are in a hurry. When we try to maintain this fast pace with our elderly facing dementia, they put on the brakes. Too much information is coming at them way too fast.

To get a better understanding, let me share with you some scientific facts on the brain. According to the article "Why It's So Hard To Pay Attention, Explained By Science" by Daniel J. Levitin (https://www.fastcompany.com/3051417/why-its-so-hard-to-pay-attention-explained-by-science): "In 2011, Americans took in five times as much information every day as they did in 1986. During our leisure time, not counting work, each of us processes approximately 100,000 words, every day."

The same article further tells us that "the processing capacity of the conscious mind has been estimated (by the researcher Mihaly Csikszentmihalyi and independently by

Bell Labs engineer Robert Lucky) at 120 bits per second. This is the speed limit for the influx of information we can pay conscious attention to at any one time.

What does this mean regarding our communication with others? To understand one person speaking to us, we need to process 60 bits of information per second. With a processing limit of 120 bits per second, this means you can barely understand two people talking to you at the same time."

To top it off, these facts are gathered on those of us whose brain is functioning at its full capacity—imagine the impact when the brain is assaulted by dementia. The ability to take in and understand information shrinks. Alzheimer's plaques and tangles eventually destroy connections in the brain, and a stroke destroys a piece of the brain in one fell swoop. Small strokes called TIAs (transient ischemic attack) which appear to resolve quickly leave the brain weakened and their effects add up over time. These all affect the way our brains receive and process information.

A person living with dementia needs more time to process the information you are presenting. It is helpful to talk slower—not so slow that you sound absurd, but slower than you normally do. Allow time to let the information be processed before expecting a response. Take a deep breath and let them move at their own pace.

Pay attention to the environment. If it is loud, busy or chaotic, the person is having to deal with all that information as well. This leaves even less capacity for conversation or completing everyday tasks. When you bring your elderly loved one to a family party, they often get exhausted quickly and may want to go home or need to go to another room where it is quiet for a bit. Their brain literally needs to rest.

If you need to get somewhere at a specific time, make sure to come early to pick them up. Take a moment to talk first and allow ample time in case they are not ready. Rushing will cause increased confusion and frustration, and they will most likely put on the brakes and stop altogether until they feel in control again.

Two Truths and a Bridge

This explains how we try to make sense of our world. A person with dementia is trying to make sense of the facts they know or believe to be true. In order for the truths to make sense, they create a scenario that ties them together.

For instance, let's say we know two truths:

#1: I have beautiful real silverware.

#2: It is missing. I can't find it.

The Bridge: Someone must have broken in during the night and stole it. In reality, the person has hidden the silverware because they heard about a burglary on the news.

We all do this in our daily life.

#1: Your employee was dressed nice today.

#2 They left early from work.

The Bridge: They are interviewing for another job. That is the assumption or bridge, where in reality, he is actually taking his wife out to dinner for their anniversary. We will respond to the assumption until we learn a new truth.

Forever Age

I coined this phrase to describe the phenomenon of holding yourself at an age range in your mind. When I hit my late 40's, I remember getting up one morning and looking in the mirror only to find my mother staring back at me. Inside I still felt like I was 30, maybe 35... but definitely not the 40-something in the mirror.

I'm sure we can all think of a time we got dressed up to the nines to go out. After you've finished your hair and makeup, you take a look in the mirror and think, "I look good!" However, when you take a picture, the darn thing doesn't show the woman you saw in the mirror! You look older. You had seen a glimpse of your forever age in the mirror, but the camera can't capture that memory. It captured you, the you of today, and that didn't fit what you saw in your mind.

I recently went to dinner with a friend, and her mother of about 80 was with us. We had taken a photo earlier in the evening. When she saw the picture, she hated it. "I don't look that old!" she declared. The photo didn't match the way she saw herself. Her forever age and the woman in the picture didn't match.

I recommend having pictures of your loved one in their 30's and 40's in photo albums and in frames in their room for them to recognize themselves. They will be great conversation starters, and you might even hear a story you have never heard before.

Chapter 6

Sandwich Generation

The term Sandwich Generation was coined in 1981 to describe adults in their 30's and 40's raising their children and caring for their parents. Today, this includes those who are moving toward their 40's to 60's. https://en.wikipedia.org/wiki/Sandwich_generation

There are 5 life balancing ideas for the caregiver:

1. Find support from a spouse, sibling, local support group or a friend—a person who will be honest and tell you when you need a break, and will then help you make it happen.

2. Take breaks and do something for yourself every day.

3. Remember the power of breathing. We often forget how important a deep breath is. Take a few long, slow deep breaths and let your thoughts fade away.

4. Be mindful of what you put into your body and get enough sleep.

5.   Ask for help when you need it, delegate what you can, and know when you can't do it anymore.

"I'm Fine."

What do you do when your parent says, "I'm fine," but you know they are not? This is a common question I get asked all the time. Here are some tips on how to assess if they really are fine.

1.   Does the house seem to be different? I.e., the rooms are not as clean as they used to be, there is an odd smell, the food in the fridge looks old.

2.   You get a sinking feeling that something isn't right. Remember, trust your intuition—it is normally right.

3.   Investigate medications.

   a.   Does the prescription bottle number of pills and dates make sense? In other words, if the prescription date is over a month old and was filled with 30 pills to be taken one time a day, but you find it with 20 pills still in it, they are not taking them as ordered and therefore not getting the benefit. Often times they report to their doctor that they are not getting better and the doctor may adjust dosages not knowing that the pills are not really being taken at all.

   b.   Are there expired medications on hand?

c.   Take medications and over the counter medications to the pharmacy to be reviewed for interactions and instructions.

d.   A medication system like a pill box or electronic dispenser may be helpful.

Brain Exercises

There are many ways to exercise the brain, and they all have something in common to hold off dementia: **they all require complete concentration.**

Rob Winningham from the Western Oregon University is known for using brain games to help the memory. He teaches that through doing activities that require a singular focus, you can postpone dementia. Playing a game of Sudoku requires you to focus on those nine numbers and how they fit into the pattern. You can't be making a mental shopping list at the same time—you have to concentrate. Professor Winningham has partnered with a company called Activity Connection to create a resource of over 200 games to stimulate the brain.

While there is still research and dispute going on about computer games to improve memory and slow down cognitive decline, it can't hurt.

In an article from the Washington Post, "Brain-training games don't really train brains" by Jenna Gallegos (https://www.washingtonpost.com/news/to-your-health/

wp/2017/07/10/brain-training-games-dont-really-train-brains-a-new-study-suggests/?utm_term=.95bc54419bcb), they dispute the effectiveness of games but also state, "Any activity that requires paying close attention flexes our ECN, and it's possible that older people may benefit from such exercises even though youthful brains don't."

Chapter 7

Music & Memories

Music is a powerful modality. Think of a song that has meaning for you. It takes you back to a specific place in time. You hear the music, feel the beat, see the memory, and relive the emotion.

The organization *musicandmemory.org* demonstrates the powerful impact that listening to music that is important to you—songs that have meaning to your life—can have on your brain. Listening to this "special" music, usually done with an iPod or similar device, awakens the whole brain for short periods. The YouTube video "Alive inside clip of Henry" shows this process in great detail.

Mini-Mental Exam

This is a common test given by a doctor or neurologist or nurse to get a baseline on cognitive status. The test is scored 0-30, with 30 being a perfect score. A score of 25-30 is considered normal. The National Institute for Health and Care

Excellence (NICE) classifies 21-24 as mild, 10-20 as moderate and <10 as severe impairment.

The test consists of a series of verbal and written questions and tasks. This includes simple questions such as, "What is the day, the year, the city you live in," and written tasks like copying a drawing or drawing a clock set at a specific time each score points. There are three words the person is asked to remember at the beginning of the test, then revisited for accuracy later in the test as well.

"Tell Me About It"

You can find this phrase used by most professionals today whose practice is with those affected by dementia. Teepa Snow has a great YouTube video demonstrating the technique, "Communicate with patient with dementia/ Alzheimer's." It can also be experienced through Improv from the University of Washington in a YouTube presentation entitled "Using Improv to improve life with Alzheimer's."

"Tell me about it" has been part of my language for as long as I can remember. I believe these are the most powerful words you can use to open up a conversation. This simple phrase allows a person to share whatever is on their mind at the time without judgement or question—it is not important if the details are true or not.

Five Minutes

Giving someone with dementia eye contact and undivided attention for just five minutes will open up conversation and connection. In today's multi-tasking, fast-paced world, we seem to have lost the importance of intentional listening. When having a conversation with someone who has dementia, you must slow down and simplify. Keep sentences short and to one subject, and give them time to respond. For example, ask them to "Tell me about the picture" while looking through a photo album, then wait for them to respond. Set aside five minutes to talk about what they share with you without interruption. Turn off the phone and all distractions. Be focused.

Chapter 8

Family Roles

In most families, there will be one person who takes the brunt of the responsibility for the care of a loved one with dementia. It is most often a daughter or daughter-in-law. On the other hand, it is common for the finances and health care decisions to be divided among family members. In this story, it is Maureen who took care of her mother while her brother, Grant, took charge of the finances.

In order to make decisions about healthcare and finances, we must learn that it is now necessary to cross boundaries that had been previously established. Finances are a topic that normally isn't discussed with children, and healthcare decisions are too often put off until an emergency forces us to consider them. This could be the case because both finances and healthcare are deeply tied to emotions.

That said, it is critical to maintain open communication with your parents before anything happens. Sit down with them and write down what their wishes are in case of a health emergency. This conversation includes far more than whether they would like CPR or not.

Personally, I always recommend talking with them at a doctor's appointment. An emergency respondent can only follow a doctor's order, so it is important to check into what your state requires and have that information readily available. This may be a difficult conversation, but it will save you from having to make a decision in the middle of an emergency. In the case that these decisions are not written down, and the family is arguing about the level of treatment they would like them to have, the one with the most aggressive care wish is followed.

Finances are often kept private and can be a touchy subject as well. If your parents want to keep this information to themselves, I would encourage them to talk to their attorney or financial advisor to protect their future. They can then state their wishes legally so they can be followed later while still keeping their privacy.

A Power of Attorney for Finances and Healthcare are good ideas to explore.

Chapter 9

Statistics

According to the Alzheimer's Association website (www.Alz.org):

- in 2018, 5.7 million Americans have been diagnosed with Alzheimer's

- 200,000 are below the age of 65

- Two-thirds of the 5.7 million are women

- Alzheimer's is the 6th leading cause of death in the United States

- Between the years of 2000 and 2015, the death rate of Alzheimer's rose by 123%

- In the same period, heart disease decreased by 11%

- One of three seniors die from a form of dementia, more than breast cancer and prostate cancer combined

Reality Orientation

Reality Orientation is when we stick to the facts.

"Today is July 2018."

"You live at this community now."

"Your husband is dead."

Growing up, you were likely taught always to tell the truth. However, in the case of someone with dementia, telling the truth is no longer the first priority. Their understanding of truth is what we follow—no matter how far from the actual truth it is.

When we challenge their understanding of truth, they feel as if we are calling them a liar, or worse—we are calling them stupid. It makes them angry, and you actually both lose.

Therapeutic Lie

There is no reason to lie to someone with dementia. We don't like to be lied to, and neither do they. We don't come across as genuine when we lie. On the other hand, a therapeutic lie is the technique of telling a lie meant to distract the person from a persistent question or statement such as "I want to go home," or "Where is my husband?" An example of a therapeutic lie is saying, "Your husband was here this morning and had to go to work. He will be back later."

The therapeutic lie is taught to those in school to become a caregiver, nurse, and even a doctor. It is a practice that some communities for those with dementia still employ, but it is not necessary. You can use so many other techniques (see below under "the hardest question") like "Tell me about it," or "What would your husband be doing at this time on a Monday?" Then we go along with what they bring up. As long as we stay with what they introduce, true or not, and we refrain from creating additional stories, we are not lying. We are joining them where they are at the moment, and that is the goal.

Accepting Emotions

We all experience a wide range of emotions. We can be happy one moment and sad the next; we can get heated and angry for a few hours and then calm down to return to a peaceful state. Emotions are a natural part of life and are meant to be felt, not just swept under the rug. It is especially important to remember this in the case of dementia.

As caregivers—as people, rather—we want to help everyone feel better. We do all we can to brighten up someone's day and cheer them up when they feel down. Accepting a hard emotion like grief or sadness is difficult.

Naomi Feil, founder of the Validation Institute, and a world-renowned speaker on dementia reminds us that we are all trying to find peace at the end of our lives. Being able to talk about our emotions and to free the hurt or loneliness we carry allows us to find some peace. It is important to face the emotion head on instead of turning away from it when it is brought to you. A family member or caregiver is called to listen without judgement and be open to what is shared with them.

The Hardest Question

Families and professionals alike struggle more with one question than all the others: when the patient is asking "Where is my husband?" after they have passed away. Families often fall back to reality orientation, telling them over and over again that Dad is gone. He died. She, hearing it again for the first time, cries. Next, they try the therapeutic lie. This time they say, "Dad is at work. He will be there later." However, he doesn't come home, and the question is asked again and again.

To face this question or the "I want to go home" to a home that no longer exists, try "Tell me about your husband. Tell me about home." Often, they have a memory that is there they need to share. It relieves the anxiety. I can almost guarantee you that they are thinking, *someone is finally listening to me.*

Another technique is to say, "It is 10 a.m. on a Monday. Where would your husband be at 10 a.m. on a Monday?" Often, they say something like, "At work, of course." Then you can ask the "Tell me about his work" question and move the conversation forward.

It takes practice, but you can do it.

Bonus Technique: You're Right - We all love to be right!

In neurolinguistics programming (NLP) we learn that when someone is ready to defend themselves, and you agree with them by saying "You're right," you confuse the brain, allowing a few seconds to introduce new information that the brain will accept. It becomes even more powerful if you can get the person to turn and walk with you in a new direction.

Example: A person with dementia stands at a door wanting to leave late at night. When you ask them to come to another room, they state, "You just want me to leave this door," ready for a battle about it. Instead of fighting, you simply reply, "You're right, and in the living room I have hot cocoa waiting for you." The "you're right" creates confusion in the brain, so they come with you into the next room and leave the door behind without argument.

I like to remind everyone I teach that the communication techniques in the book are not rocket science; they are simple and easy to use with practice. They also work with spouses, children, and friends. Communication is complex—we can use all the reminders we can get.

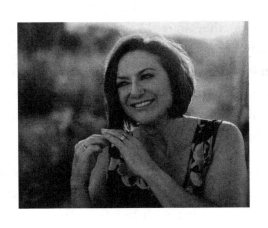

About the Author

Angelia Brigance had the privilege of growing up with her grandparents. As a result, she was able to truly understand the gift that the elderly are to us and the importance of treating them with dignity, respect, and love. This understanding grew into a passion for helping the senior community thrive, with a focus on helping people understand and communicate with those who have dementia. She uses her heart for Seniors to fuel herself to continue to be a leader in the senior community.

For the last 26 years, Angelia's career has been focused on navigating the many challenges that seniors face. In addition to her years of on-the-job experience, she has an Associates Degree in Developmental Disabilities, a Bachelor's Degree in Psychology, and a Masters of Science in Counseling. She has also successfully completed studies in Geriatrics, Validation, and Neurolinguistic Programming. Angelia's experience and education allow her to successfully coach and train professionals, families, and businesses in the senior world.

Angelia is a member of the Washington Athletic Club Speakers Bureau and is published in their magazine. She has also been published in other local magazines on issues affecting seniors and was interviewed on *New Day Northwest*. She has taught communications, conflict resolution, and leadership skills for a variety of companies, including Starbucks. Most recently she was a guest teacher at Northwest University.

In the last few years, Angelia has survived a ruptured brain aneurysm and Stage 3 Lung Cancer, which has motivated her now more than ever to help others feel gratitude and optimism in the face of their own personal life challenges. Angelia is married with two adult children, one grandson, and enjoys spending the weekends hiking with her husband and two dogs.